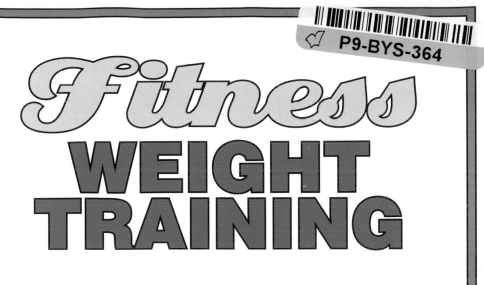

Fitness
WEIGHT
TRAINING

FITNESS SPECTRUM SERIES

Thomas R. Baechle
Roger W. Earle

Creighton University
Omaha, Nebraska

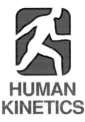

HUMAN
KINETICS

Library of Congress Cataloging-in-Publication Data

Baechle, Thomas R., 1943-
    Fitness weight training / Tom R. Baechle, Roger W. Earle.
      p. cm. -- (Fitness spectrum series)
    Includes index.
    ISBN 0-87322-445-0
    1. Weight training. 2. Physical fitness. I. Earle, Roger W.,
1967-   . II. Series.
    GV546.B33 1995   94-28361
    613.7'13--dc20   CIP

ISBN: 0-87322-445-0

Copyright © 1995 by Human Kinetics Publishers, Inc.

Developmental Editor: Marni Basic; **Assistant Editors:** Ed Giles, Julie Lancaster, Julie Ohnemus, John Wentworth; **Copyeditor:** Anthony Brown; **Proofreader:** Myla Smith; **Indexer:** Theresa J. Schaefer; **Typesetter:** Ruby Zimmerman; **Text Designer:** Keith Blomberg; **Layout Artist:** Stuart Cartwright; **Cover Designer:** Jack Davis; **Photographer (cover):** Ray Malace; **Photographer (interior):** Chris Brown; **Illustrators:** Beth Young, Thomas-Bradley Illustration, Studio 2D, Keith Blomberg; **Printer:** Bang Printing

Human Kinetics books are available at special discounts for bulk purchase. Special editions or book excerpts can also be created to specification. For details, contact the Special Sales Manager at Human Kinetics.

Printed in the United States of America   10 9 8 7 6 5 4 3 2 1

Human Kinetics
P.O. Box 5076, Champaign, IL 61825-5076
1-800-747-4457

Canada: Human Kinetics, Box 24040, Windsor, ON N8Y 4Y9
1-800-465-7301 (in Canada only)

Europe: Human Kinetics, P.O. Box IW14, Leeds LS16 6TR, England
(44) 532 781708

Australia: Human Kinetics, 2 Ingrid Street, Clapham 5062, South Australia
(08) 371 3755

New Zealand: Human Kinetics, P.O. Box 105-231, Auckland 1
(09) 309 2259

We walk through this life but once. Thus, we are challenged to maximize our energy and talents in ways that will make the greatest contributions to others. This book provides us a vehicle for communicating to thousands information that might improve the quality of their lives.

Writing this book has provided yet another opportunity for us as close friends to acquire greater respect and admiration for each other's talents. It also has given us the chance to reflect on and appreciate the significant and positive impact our families and special friends have had on our lives. We dedicate this book to them:

Acknowledgments

There are some special people who made this book a reality and to whom we are indebted. Those individuals include Ted Miller, director of the HK Trade Division, and Marni Basic, developmental editor. Both provided invaluable insight concerning the direction of this book. We are also indebted to the many other professionals at Human Kinetics who have contributed their expertise. Lastly we are fortunate to have had the support and keyboarding skills of Linda Tranisi, Kim Johnson, Ryan Schmitz, Olga Ortega, and Kelli Watson throughout the process of completing this book.

Contents

Credits

Selected data in the Bench Press Test on page 25 and the Muscular Fitness Norms (Bench Press) table on page 26 were obtained from *Y's Way to Fitness*, by J.A. Golding, C.R. Meyers, and W.E. Sinning, 1991, Chicago: National Board of YMCA.

The stretch descriptions on pages 36 to 39 are from *Weight Training: Steps to Success* (pp. 18-19, 146) by T.R. Baechle and B.R. Groves, 1992, Champaign, IL: Leisure Press. Copyright 1992 by Leisure Press. Adapted by permission of Human Kinetics.

Tables 12.2, 12.8, 12.9, and 12.10 are from *Weight Training: Steps to Success* (pp. 43, 135, 136) by T.R. Baechle and B.R. Groves, 1992, Champaign, IL: Leisure Press. Copyright 1992 by Leisure Press. Reprinted by permission of Human Kinetics.

PART I

PREPARING TO WEIGHT TRAIN

Weight training is taking fitness enthusiasts by storm, and it has even become attractive to thousands who once would have called themselves couch potatoes. It's an activity that can be done in a short period, yet it makes dramatic changes in how your body looks and feels. Many who weight train would tell you that having a firm body not only feels great—it also positively affects how you relate to others, increases your energy level, and improves your productivity at work and in many everyday activities.

Weight training helps to maintain muscle strength, muscular endurance, neuromuscular (nerve-muscle) coordination, and bone density (helping to avoid osteoporosis). The latest research suggests that weight training makes a significant contribution to quality of life, whatever one's age or gender.

No matter what your weight training experience is, you'll find helpful information in this book. If you have little or no experience weight training, we'll provide the basics to get you started. If you've trained before but without much organization to your approach, you'll benefit from the guidance offered by the structured programs. If you have a great deal of weight training experience, we'll show you how to train better and get more from your workouts.

The upcoming part of the book begins by describing the three different types of training outcomes that structure the workouts in Part II. The remaining chapters in Part I lay the groundwork for your weight training and will help you get the most out of each session, including:

- Understanding how weight training's physical benefits compare to those of other activities
- Determining what weight training equipment to use, where to train, and how to choose and buy equipment
- Assessing your weight training fitness level to help determine where to start and how intensely to train
- Executing exercises safely
- Warming up, stretching, and cooling down properly

1

Weight Training for Fitness

"Another weight training book? Forget it! There are hundreds already available." That was our reaction when we were asked to write *Fitness Weight Training*, and it may be yours when you first pick it up.

But this book is different. It's not the typical how-to manual. You won't find exhaustive explanations of how to perform exercises; nor will you find technical anatomical or physiological information that is difficult to understand.

Fitness Weight Training is a book you can use immediately, because it provides a compilation of color-coded workouts that are easy to understand and use. It will quickly become your new workout companion and your weight room guide to success!

No matter what your weight training appetite or fitness level may be, you'll find something here to satisfy you. The workouts range from easy, short ones for the beginner to intense, more lengthy sessions for the highly trained. Best of all, *Fitness Weight Training* is designed to match your individual tastes. The individual workouts are structured around three different outcomes: muscle toning (to tone up muscles), body shaping (to develop larger muscles and shape your body), and strength training (to significantly improve your strength).

Muscle Toning

Toned muscles exhibit a tight or firm appearance, versus a loose or flabby one. They are also defined, which means you can see distinct muscle separations, indentations, and shapes—in other words, muscles that are not smooth in appearance.

Muscle toning is a natural outcome of regular weight training. If you are interested in muscle toning, higher repetitions in your training will produce better muscle tone qualities without large increases in muscle size. Therefore, the result of following a muscle toning program will be firmer, harder, and more defined muscles without significant muscle size increases.

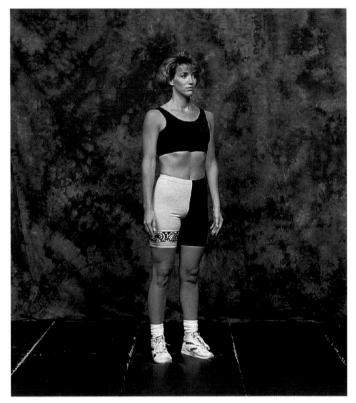

A muscle toned body.

Body Shaping

Body shaping programs provide all of the same benefits associated with muscle toning programs, but they also increase the size of muscles more dramatically. With body shaping you'll not only experience the muscle firming and definition of muscle toning, you will increase your muscle size.

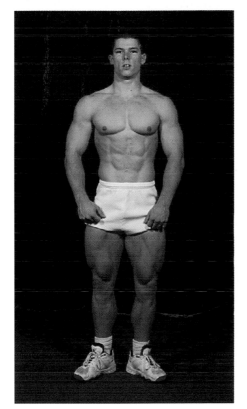

A body shaped body.

Strength Training

Strength is the muscle's ability to exert force. Typically, the term strength is associated with the ability to exert maximum force during a single effort, sometimes referred to as a one repetition maximum effort (1RM). For instance, let's say you loaded the bar to 100 pounds and were told to perform as many repetitions as possible. If you could do only one repetition, your **1 R**(epetition) **M**(aximum) or **1RM**, would equal 100 pounds. Strength increases can make major contributions to recreational and competitive sports performances as well as make everyday tasks—regardless of age—a lot easier. Strength training programs usually produce muscle size gains greater than toning programs but not to the same extent that a body shaping program will.

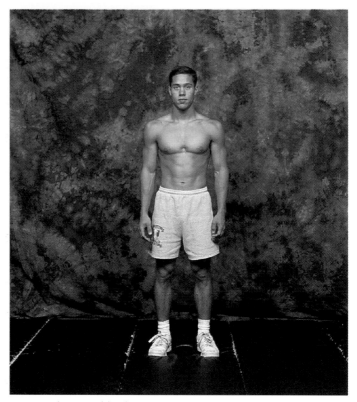

A strength trained body.

Why Not Walk or Jog Instead?

Aerobic exercises such as walking and jogging are ideal for improving cardiovascular fitness and improving muscular endurance in the legs, but these activities contribute little to shaping your body and to improving your overall flexibility, muscular endurance, and strength levels in the upper body. The advantage of aerobic activities over weight training is that they require minimal equipment and you can do them almost anywhere. Swimming, cycling, and cross-country skiing, which are also aerobic activities, contribute better than walking or jogging to overall flexibility, muscular endurance, and strength, but they still fall short of what weight training programs do for strengthening and shaping specific areas of the body. As you can see in the chart on page 7, weight training programs improve muscular strength, endurance, body composition (ratio of muscle and fat to total body weight), flexibility, and to a much lesser extent, cardiovascular fitness. So, if your goal is to improve cardiovascular fitness, you should include one or more of the aerobic types of exercise mentioned in your training program. But if your goal is to improve your overall flexibility, muscular endurance, strength, and body composition, then you've picked the right type of exercise and the right book!

How weight training compares to other fitness activities.

Unlike other exercise activities that rely on developing specific muscles (for example, walking and cycling primarily develop the legs), weight training programs can be designed to develop the legs as well as many other muscle groups—especially those that are particularly important to you. Weight training is like going through a cafeteria and picking which foods you want to eat, instead of having to eat simply what they serve you. The workouts presented in chapters 6 through 11 of this book emphasize exercises for seven major muscle groups (chest, back, shoulders, arms— front and back, abdomen, and legs) but also include those for the forearm, calf, and neck.

How well your program is designed and how diligently you follow it will determine how successfully you achieve your desired outcome. What makes weight training exciting is the rapid rate at which you can see and feel changes in your body! As soon as you start exercising, your muscles feel firmer, and the "body sculpting" process begins. Regular training will convince you that you have the ability to shape your body in attractive ways that you may never have expected!

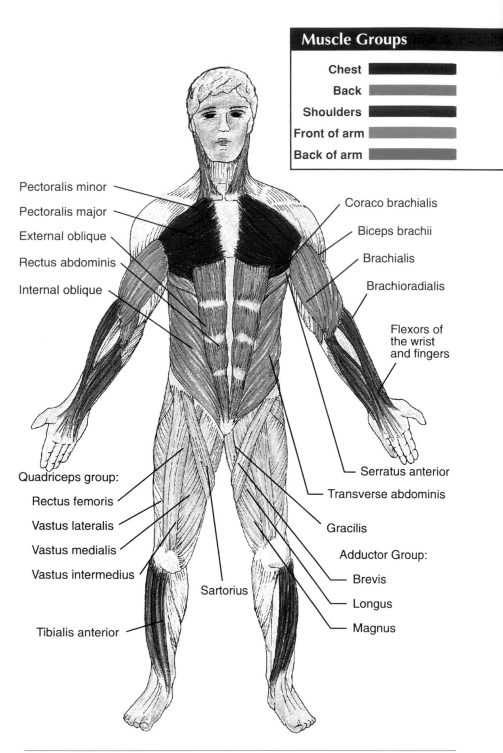

Muscle Groups

Chest	▬▬▬
Back	▬▬▬
Shoulders	▬▬▬
Front of arm	▬▬▬
Back of arm	▬▬▬

Pectoralis minor

Pectoralis major

External oblique

Rectus abdominis

Internal oblique

Coraco brachialis

Biceps brachii

Brachialis

Brachioradialis

Flexors of the wrist and fingers

Quadriceps group:

Rectus femoris

Vastus lateralis

Vastus medialis

Vastus intermedius

Sartorius

Serratus anterior

Transverse abdominis

Gracilis

Adductor Group:

Brevis

Longus

Magnus

Tibialis anterior

Muscles, front view.

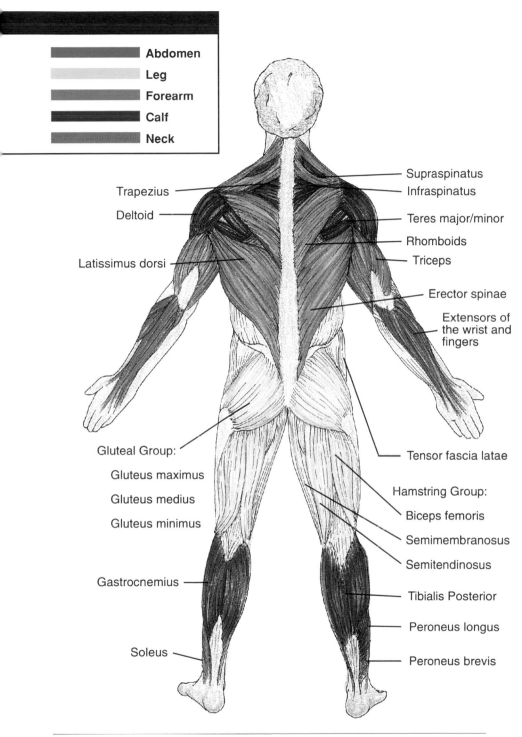

Abdomen
Leg
Forearm
Calf
Neck

Supraspinatus
Infraspinatus
Trapezius
Deltoid
Teres major/minor
Rhomboids
Latissimus dorsi
Triceps
Erector spinae
Extensors of the wrist and fingers
Gluteal Group:
Gluteus maximus
Gluteus medius
Gluteus minimus
Tensor fascia latae
Hamstring Group:
Biceps femoris
Semimembranosus
Semitendinosus
Gastrocnemius
Tibialis Posterior
Peroneus longus
Peroneus brevis
Soleus

Muscles, rear view.

2

Getting Equipped

What weight training equipment to use, what to wear, and how to identify a suitable place to train and qualified people to teach you are not common knowledge. This chapter will inform you in all of these areas so that you can get equipped with confidence!

Weight Training Equipment

Weight training equipment falls into two major categories: machines and free weights. Both types are typically used in schools, colleges, health clubs, and corporate settings; free weight equipment is the most common choice for home training.

Machines

The two most common types of weight training machines are pivot machines (single- and multi-unit) and cam machines.

Pivot Machines (PM). Pivot machines have one or more stacks of weights that are lifted by pulling or pushing a weight arm attached to a pivot point. Single-unit machines are designed to work one muscle area, whereas multi-unit machines have various stations that let you work many muscle areas by moving from station to station. Pivot machines have both fixed pivot and moving pivot designs, and many multi-unit machines use both.

Fixed-resistance pivot machines have one or more fixed weight stacks that are lifted by pulling or pushing a weight arm attached to a fixed pivot point. The limitation of this type of equipment is that at some points during the exercise the load does not tax the muscles as much as others. As a result, different positions require more effort than others, as though someone were changing the load during each repetition.

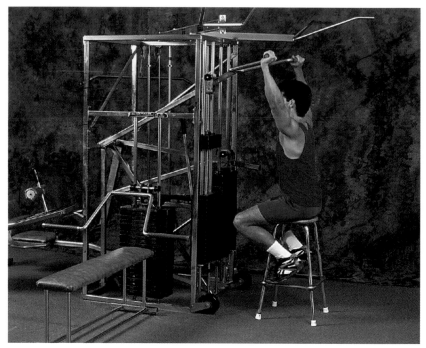

A multi-unit pivot machine.

Like the fixed-resistance machine, the variable-resistance pivot machine also has a weight arm attached to a pivot point. But the weight stack moves or rolls back and forth on a weight arm, allowing a more consistent load on muscles. When the weight arm moves to a position that would require less effort, the weight stack slides to a position requiring more effort. Conversely, when the weight arm moves to a position that would require more effort, the weight stack moves to a position requiring less effort.

Cam Machines (CM).   A cam machine is a variable-resistance machine that features an elliptically shaped wheel, referred to as a cam. Its shape makes the cam function similarly to a moving weight stack. As the chain (cable or belt) tracks over the peaks and valleys of the cam, the distance between the point of rotation (the axle on which the cam rotates) and the weight stack varies to produce a more consistent load on the muscles.

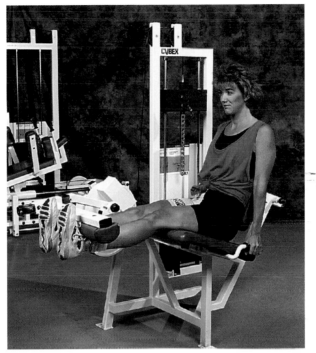

A cam machine.

SAFETY CONSIDERATIONS FOR MACHINES

Weight training machines are considered by many to be safer than free weight equipment because the weight stack is positioned so that it cannot fall off or fall on you. Also, machine exercises typically do not require the same degree of muscular coordination as free weight exercises. Another advantage is that machine exercises can be performed without a spotter. With that said, do not think for a minute that you cannot be seriously injured on a machine. There are probably more machine- than free weight–related injuries reported each year. By developing an understanding of how to properly use machines (as discussed in chapter 12), you will find them to be a very safe and time-efficient type of weight training equipment.

Free Weight Equipment

Free weights—barbells and dumbbells—cost less than weight machines and offer tremendous versatility, making your choice of exercises virtually unlimited.

Barbells. Barbells are used in two-arm exercises. The typical barbell has a middle section that includes both smooth and knurled (roughened) areas with collars on each side. The weight plates slide up to the collars to stop them from sliding inward toward the hands. The outside collars, sometimes referred to as locks, slide up to the plates and keep them from sliding off the ends of the bar. A 6-foot bar with collars and locks weighs approximately 30 pounds (5 pounds per foot of the bar). Cambered or curl bars have the same characteristics as standard bars except the curves enable you to isolate certain muscle groups better than when using a straight bar.

At training facilities you will usually find 6-foot standard and cambered bars and 7-foot Olympic bars. Olympic bars have the same diameter as most bars except for the section between the collar and the end of the bar where the diameter is greater. Olympic bars are heavier than their standard counterparts, weighing 45 pounds without locks. Olympic weight plates, which have larger holes than standard weight plates, are designed for use only with the Olympic bar.

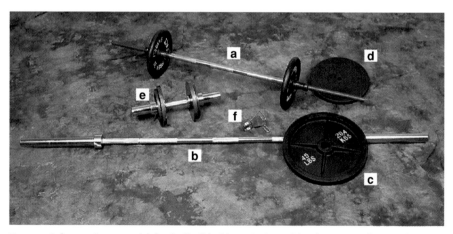

Free weight equipment: (a) barbell; (b) Olympic bar; (c) Olympic style weight plate; (d) standard weight plate; (e) standard dumbbell; (f) standard lock.

Dumbbells. Dumbbells are used in one- and two-arm exercises. Though they are sometimes premolded, it is more common in training facilities to see dumbbells designed similarly to barbells. Dumbbells are shorter than barbells and their entire middle section (between weight plates) is usually knurled. A dumbbell bar with collars and locks weighs approximately 3 pounds. Usually only the weight of the plates is considered when the weight of the dumbbell is recorded. For example, a dumbbell with a 10-pound plate on either side is listed as weighing 20, not 23, pounds.

SAFETY CONSIDERATIONS FOR FREE WEIGHTS

The term "free" in free weight means that the equipment does not restrict joint movement. As a result, using free weight barbells and dumbbells requires a higher level of muscle coordination than using machines. Because of this freedom of movement, injuries are more likely to occur when you don't use correct loading, lifting, and spotting techniques. When reasonable precautions are taken (as discussed in chapter 4), free weight training is very safe, and it can be more fun than machines while also being more effective in strengthening joint structures.

Weight Training Attire

There is really no standard type of weight training attire. You will see everything from tight-fitting, one-piece suits (similar to those worn by wrestlers) to baggy pants and shirts. Men often wear tank tops or T-shirts, shorts, and gym shoes. Women may wear these or choose to wear shorts over a bodysuit.

Beyond the clothes on your back, it's a good idea to give special attention to several other important areas.

Gloves

Weight training gloves are not a necessity, but they will help you avoid the development of calluses and will provide you with a better grip. Purchase flexible gloves that fit your hands snugly.

Shoes

Wear shoes that have good lateral support. Look for shoes that have a normal-sized heel width, such as tennis shoes, rather than the wide or waffle heel on jogging shoes. Cross-training shoes are a good choice over those designed for aerobic dance, but both are suitable.

Weight Belts

Another type of gear seen in weight rooms is a 4- to 6-inch-wide belt made of leather or nylon. Weight belts add support to the lower back, especially during overhead lifting or heavy squatting exercises.

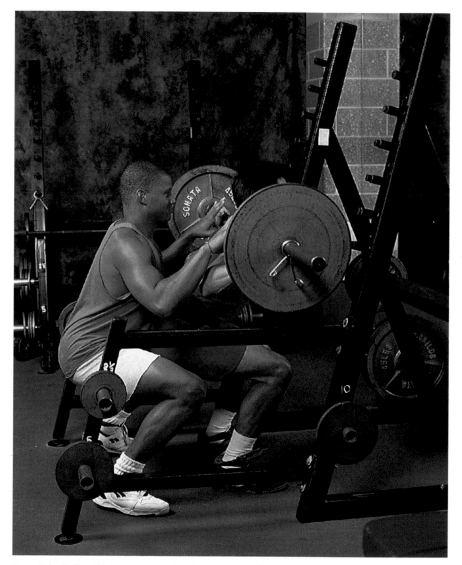

A weight belt adds support to the lower back during overhead lifting or heavy squatting exercises.

Other Supportive Equipment

Other supportive equipment that you might use are wraps worn on the knees, elbows, and/or wrists. Usually they are made of elastic, but they may also be made of neoprene, cotton strips, or leather. Wraps create warmth and are sometimes used to provide additional stabilization of joints. They should not be used to compensate for unstable joints, unless recommended by a physician.

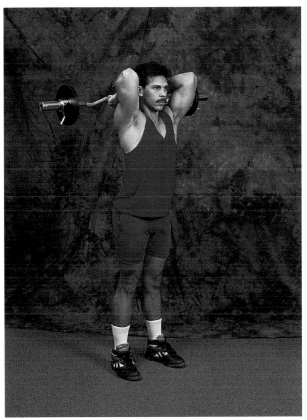

There is no "typical" weight training attire. Wear clothing you're comfortable in.

What Not to Wear

Before you enter the weight room, take care to remove any items that may cause injury. Earrings, necklaces, watches, and rings can catch on equipment and get ripped off, smashed, or create abrasions and cuts.

ADDING UP THE COSTS: ATTIRE AND SUPPORTIVE EQUIPMENT

Here are the approximate costs of the equipment previously discussed, all of which can be purchased at most sporting goods stores.

ITEM	WOMEN	MEN
BODY SUIT	$ 30-50	$ ——
GLOVES	10-15	10-15
WEIGHT BELT	20-90	20-90
SHOES	50-150	50-150
SHORTS	20	20
TANK TOP	15	15
TOTAL COST:	$ 145-340	$ 115-290

Where Will You Train?

You can weight train in one of two places: in your home or at a fitness facility. The following sections discuss the pros and cons of each option.

Training at Home

For many, training at home is the only practical option because of time constraints, cost of a fitness facility membership, or both. Many people simply prefer to train in the quiet of their own homes. If you want to train at home, there are several basic equipment and space issues to consider.

Where to Train at Home. Begin by determining a suitable area for training as well as storing equipment. It should be out of the main "travel routes" in your home; it should be well ventilated, well lighted, have at least one electrical outlet; and it should be securable (if you have young children). An electrical outlet offers the opportunity to plug in a stereo, radio, or maybe a treadmill or stair stepper. If you have a choice, select an area that has a high ceiling. Be sure to position equipment away from doors.

Avoid working out on tile floors or concrete because tile is slippery and both are easily damaged when dropping barbells and dumbbells and moving equipment. Carpet-covered concrete provides a better training surface. A plywood lifting platform can also be used. The ideal floor is a rubberized surface (one-quarter-inch or more thick), but this is a very expensive option.

Basic Equipment Requirements. The minimum amount and types of equipment you need to use when following a basic weight program consists of a standard barbell with collars and locks, a set of adjustable dumbbells, 80 pounds of standard weight plates, and a bench press. Those intending to follow a more aggressive program should purchase an additional 135 pounds of weight plates.

For more serious lifters, basic equipment needs include an Olympic bar and locks, a set of dumbbells, 255 pounds of Olympic weight plates, and a free weight bench press designed for an Olympic bar.

You should also consider purchasing a set of squat racks. Keep in mind that both bench and squat rack exercises require one or more spotters. Weight plate and barbell storage racks are optional but nice to have.

ADDING UP THE COSTS: TRAINING AT HOME

If you plan to outfit a home weight room, plan to spend about $200 for flooring and/or the materials to construct a lifting platform. How much you spend on basic weight training equipment depends on the type of bar, the number of pounds (or kilos), and the amount of equipment you feel you need.

- 110-pound standard barbell set $150–$275
  (6-foot bar, locks, and 80 pounds of standard weight plates)
- Free weight bench press designed for a standard bar $150–$275
- Standard 310-pound Olympic barbell set $175–$300
  (7-foot bar, locks, and 255 pounds of Olympic weight plates)
- Free weight bench press designed for an Olympic bar $250–$350
- Additional items:
  Dumbbell bar (star lock) = $11.99
  Dumbbell bar (standard lock) = $6.99
  Squat rack = $369
  Bar rack = $150
  Dumbbell rack (short/long) = $119/$189
  Weight plate rack = $60

Training at a Fitness Facility

Selecting a fitness facility that will meet your needs is a challenge. If you need the expertise of a qualified trainer to help you get started, then that should be the number one criterion when deciding on where you will work out. Ideally, the facility you choose will have both qualified personnel and a wide variety of equipment and programs to meet your training needs.

Training With a Personal Trainer. A well-qualified personal trainer who understands how to motivate you can make every training day a fun and rewarding experience. A truly qualified trainer will probably have earned one or more certifications associated with the health and fitness profession. Look for someone who has received certification from the Certified Strength and Conditioning Specialist Agency, the certifying body of the National Strength and Conditioning Association (certified strength and conditioning specialist and/or NSCA-certified personal trainer); the American Council on Exercise (personal trainer); the American College of Sports Medicine (health fitness instructor); or other respected fitness-related professional organizations.

Be sure that you obtain a referral from individuals you trust—or at least observe the personal trainer in action before making a decision. How well a trainer is able to make technical information understandable is essential to your success. A good trainer will help you understand what you are doing and why you are doing it. And it never hurts to work with someone who has a motivating personality that will energize you to stick to your training program. Look for experienced trainers, because those who have been trainers for many years probably have been successful motivators and have fulfilled the needs of their clients.

Training Without a Personal Trainer. If you are new to weight training and decide to train on your own, one of your first decisions concerns whether to use weight machines or free weights. While free weights offer you the tremendous versatility of choosing among many possible exercises, they require more skill. Although machines are not foolproof, they are generally easier and safer, once you have been shown how to properly use them. Take special care when selecting loads, because sometimes even the lightest weight plate or bar may exceed your strength in a particular exercise. Also, keep in mind that the dimensions of some machines may not accommodate your physique; this is especially true for those individuals who are short, tall, or very heavy. For these reasons, it is wise to get instruction from a qualified professional for at least the first couple of weeks, because he or she can teach you how to engage in proper exercise movement patterns and how to make necessary load plate and machine adjustments. If you decide to use free weights, obtaining professional instruction is even more important.

ADDING UP THE COSTS: TRAINING AT A FITNESS FACILITY

When discussing membership contracts, pay special attention to the services that are offered a la carte, that is, at additional cost.

Single membership costs
Initiation fee $70–$250
Yearly fee $275–$580

Family membership costs
Initiation fee $85–$300
Yearly fee $345–$670

Personal trainer costs

$25–$150 per hour
Cost depends on the credentials of the trainer, services rendered, and your geographic location.

3

Checking Your Weight Training Fitness Level

Once you decide to begin an exercise program, it's natural to want to do too much too soon. If you're out of shape, remember you didn't get that way in a couple of days. Regardless of what you do, you can't get back into shape in a couple of days either, so don't try! Your attempts to do so might lead to excessive muscle soreness, extreme fatigue, less enthusiasm about resuming training, and possible injury. Use the following readiness checklist to determine if you should consult with a physician before you begin working out.

ASSESSING YOUR PHYSICAL READINESS

You should consult a physician before beginning a weight training program if you answer yes to any of the following questions.

Yes   No

____ ____ Are you over age 50 (female) or 40 (male) and not accustomed to exercise?

____ ____ Do you have a history of heart disease?

____ ____ Has a doctor ever said your blood pressure was too high?

____ ____ Are you taking any prescription medications, such as those for heart problems or high blood pressure?

____ ____ Have you ever experienced chest pain, spells of severe dizziness, or fainting?

____ ____ Do you have a history of respiratory problems, such as asthma?

____ ____ Have you had surgery or experienced bone, muscle, tendon, or ligament problems (especially back or knee) that might be aggravated by an exercise program?

____ ____ Is there a good physical or health reason not already mentioned why you should not follow a weight training program?

Test Your Weight Training Fitness

Knowing your fitness level will enable you to select a training zone that matches your current abilities and will help you to establish reasonable goals. Determine your current fitness level for weight training by using the following bench press test. The results of this test will give you a general idea of your readiness to begin weight training. Refer to pages 150 to 151 in Appendix A for an illustration of how to correctly perform the bench press.

BENCH PRESS TEST

Equipment
35-pound barbell for women
80-pound barbell for men
Flat bench press bench (with uprights)
  or
A bench press station on a single- or multi-unit machine

Directions
1. Seek the help of a qualified individual to spot for you (if you are using free weights).
2. Lie on your back with your head, shoulders, upper back, and buttocks on the bench and your feet straddled and flat on the floor.
3. With the palms up, grip the bar at a position slightly wider than shoulder width.
4. With the spotter's assistance, move the bar upward and away from the uprights until your elbows are fully extended and the bar is directly above the nipples.
5. Lower the bar to the chest and pause.
6. Push the bar upward to a full-elbow extension to complete the first repetition, and then return the bar to the chest and immediately press it again.
7. Continue pressing and lowering until you cannot complete another repetition.
8. Record the number of repetitions you complete.

Important!
Perform each repetition in a slow and controlled manner. Allow 1 to 2 seconds for pushing the bar to the extended-elbow position and 1 to 2 seconds for the downward movement to the chest. It should take 2 to 4 seconds to complete each repetition. Do not bounce the bar off the chest. As the repetitions become harder to complete, remember to breathe out when pushing upward and inhale during downward movements.

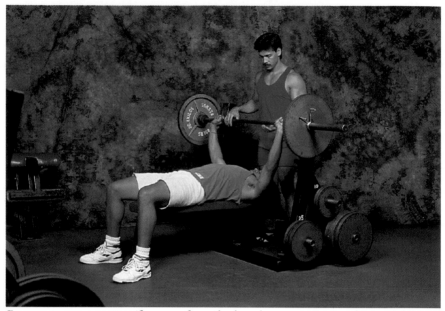

Be sure to use a spotter if you perform the bench press test using free weights.

To determine your score, refer to the top half of the table below if you are male and the lower half if you are female. Identify the appropriate age-range column, and below it find the number of repetitions you completed. At the far left column you'll find your weight training fitness level.

Now that you have determined your fitness level, you are probably eager to begin training, but you should wait until you have read each of the chapters in this part. Each of them provides essential information that will enable you to maximize every minute of training.

Muscular Fitness Norms (Bench Press)						
Fitness for weight training based on completed repetitions						
Age	18-25	26-35	36-45	46-55	56-65	66-75
			Men			
High	≥30	≥26	≥24	≥20	≥14	≥10
Average	21-29	18-25	15-23	10-19	7-13	5-9
Low	≤20	≤17	≤14	≤9	≤6	≤4
			Women			
High	≥28	≥25	≥21	≥20	≥16	≥12
Average	18-27	15-24	12-20	10-19	8-15	5-11
Low	≤17	≤14	≤11	≤9	≤7	≤4

4

Weight Training the Right Way

There is more to weight training than simply finding a barbell and "pumping iron." This chapter outlines some dos and don'ts that will let you get the most out of the time and effort you devote to training and do it safely.

Performing Exercises Correctly

The techniques of lifting involve focusing on four things: having a good grip; having a stable position from which to lift; keeping the object being lifted close to your body; and learning to use your legs, not your back, to lift.

Gripping the Bar

There are two factors to consider when establishing a grip: the *type* of grip that should be used and *how far apart* the hands should grip the bar.

Type of Grip. The grips that may be used to lift a bar off the floor are the pronated, or *overhand*, grip; the supinated, or *underhand*, grip; and the mixed, or *alternate*, grip. In the overhand grip the knuckles face up and the thumbs are toward each other. In the underhand grip, the palms face up and the thumbs face away from each other. In the alternate grip, one hand is in an underhand grip and the other in an overhand grip; the thumbs point in the same direction.

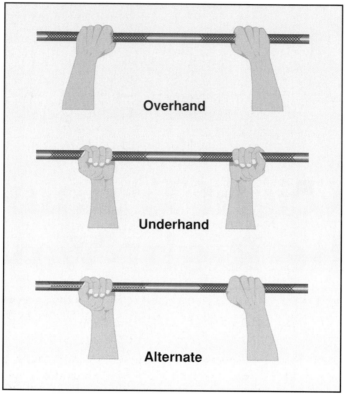

Bar grips.

All of these grips are termed closed grips, meaning that the fingers and thumbs are wrapped (closed) around the bar. In an open grip, sometimes referred to as a false grip, the thumbs do not wrap around the bar. The open grip can be very dangerous, because the bar may roll off the palms of the hand and onto the face or foot, causing severe injury. Always use a closed grip!

Width of Grip.   There are several grip widths used in weight training. In some exercises the hands are placed at about shoulder width, at an equal distance from the weight plates. This is referred to as the common grip. Some exercises require a narrower grip than this, others wider. When using Appendix A, be sure you note the type of grip and the proper width for each exercise as well as how to establish a balanced grip on the bar.

Become familiar with the smooth and knurled areas of the bar and place your hands appropriately. Incorrectly placed hands can create an imbalanced grip and result in serious injury.

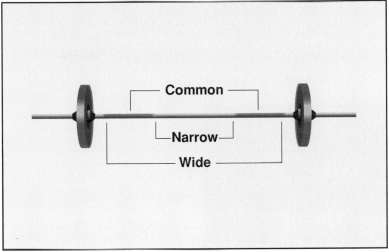

Grip widths.

Lifting the Bar

Lifting the bar correctly is important to your safety. Improper lifting places substantial stress on the lower back and can result in serious back injuries. Always observe these keys to proper lifting:

- Position your feet flat on the floor, shoulder-width apart with toes pointing slightly outward. (Establishing a stable base of support is especially important for overhead exercises with dumbbells or barbells.)
- Position your shoulders over the bar, keeping your head up and your eyes looking straight ahead.
- Establish the "flat back" position, which makes your legs, instead of your lower back, move the load.
- As you lift, think "Keep the bar close, the hips low, and the back flat."

The photo sequence on pages 30 to 31 shows how to lift the bar safely. The preparatory lifting position (frames a and b) places the body in a stable position, one in which the legs—not the back—do the lifting. Getting into the proper position is not as easy as you might think. As you squat down, one or both heels will tend to lift up, causing you to step forward to catch your balance. Remember, keep your heels on the floor! If a mirror is available, watch yourself as you squat down into the low preparatory position. Does your back stay in a flat position, and do your heels stay in contact with the floor? They should. The most important point to remember when you lift a barbell, dumbbell, weight plate, or any object off the floor is to use your *leg* muscles, not your *back* muscles.

If you need to pull the barbell to your shoulders, continue pulling it past your thighs (frames a-c); do not allow the bar to rest on your thighs. As you straighten your legs, your hips should move forward quickly, followed by a rapid shoulder shrug. In order to effectively and safely pull the bar from the thighs to the shoulders, visualize yourself jumping with the barbell while keeping your elbows straight, and at the very peak of the jump, see yourself shrugging your shoulders and flexing your elbows to catch the bar on the shoulders, as shown in frame d. Time the catch of the bar onto your shoulders so that the knees and hips are flexed as the bar makes shoulder contact (frame e).

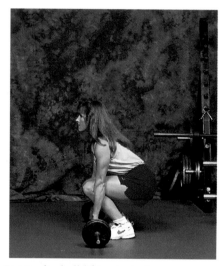

Returning the Bar to the Floor

When lowering the bar or any heavy object to the floor, remember to keep the bar or weight close to you and to keep your back flat, relying on your legs to move the bar in a slow, controlled manner to the floor.

Proper barbell lifting technique:
(a) beginning position;

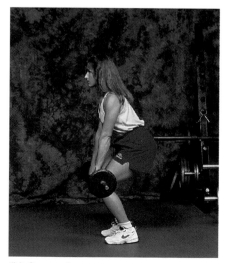

(b) first pull;

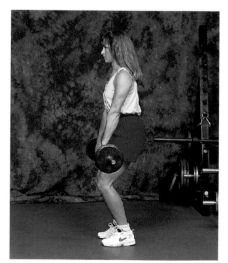

(c) scoop;

If the bar is at shoulder height, allow the bar's weight to slowly pull your arms to a straightened position, which should place the bar in a resting position (briefly) on your thighs. Hold the bar briefly at midthigh before lowering it to the floor. Remember to keep your head up and your back flat throughout the bar's return to the floor.

Using a Weight Belt

Should you wear a weight belt? The answer depends on which exercise you are performing and the amount of weight you are using. You do *not* need a belt for exercises that do not stress the back (e.g., biceps curl, lat pull-down) or for those exercises that do stress the back but involve the use of light loads (e.g., squats, overhead press). You should definitely wear a belt when performing exercises that stress the back and involve the use of maximum or near-maximum loads. When using a belt, pull it snugly around you. And remember, the use of a weight belt in and of itself *will not* protect you from back injuries—good technique will!

Breathing

Correct breathing involves breathing out during the working or sticking phase of exercise and inhaling during the relaxation phase. When lifting a bar (or other object), exhale as you pass through the most difficult part. For example, if you are lifting a bar only to thigh level, the "sticking point" would be located just above your knees. If you are pulling the bar to your shoulders, the sticking point occurs at the peak of your shoulder shrug. Remember to inhale as you lower the bar back to the floor. You will have

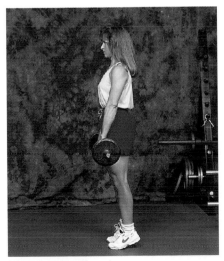

(d) second pull;

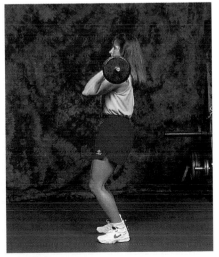

(e) catch.

a tendency to hold your breath throughout the entire exertion phase—avoid this, because it is dangerous! If you don't exhale, you reduce the return of blood to your heart and brain. And if your brain is deprived of oxygen-rich blood, you can become dizzy, and you may faint. Holding your breath is inappropriate and is especially dangerous when performing overhead exercises. Furthermore, it is even more dangerous if you have high blood pressure. Put simply, proper breathing is imperative during the execution of each exercise.

Training Precautions—Free Weights

The following precautions will make training safer and more effective by helping you avoid potentially dangerous situations.

Load Bars Properly

Take great care to load bars evenly and with the proper amount of load. If the ends of a suspended bar (on the flat or incline bench and on the squat rack supports) are not loaded evenly, the bar may tip, possibly resulting in injury. Learning to recognize the weight of different bars and of weight plates will help you in loading the bar evenly and in placing the proper amount of load on the bar.

Lock Barbells and Dumbbells

Lifting with unlocked barbells and dumbbells is dangerous. Weight plates that are not secured with locks can easily slide off the bar and land on your feet or other body parts. Before each set of exercises, locks should be checked for tightness. Do not assume that the last person using the barbell or dumbbell tightened the locks.

Avoid Backing Into Others

Take care to avoid backing into others, because an untimely bump may cause a barbell or dumbbell to fall on the head (from a standing press) or face (as in the supine dumbbell fly exercise) of someone training nearby.

Be Aware of Extended Bars

Extended bars are those that overhang or extend outward from machines, from barbells supported on racks (e.g., on the squat rack), from uprights (as for the bench press), or from bars held in the hands. Pay special attention to bars that are positioned at or above shoulder height; serious facial injuries can result from walking into bars, so be careful! The lat pull-down bar and the barbells held at or above shoulder height are likely sources of facial injuries to those who are not alert, so be especially cautious with these bars and around people who are performing overhead exercises.

Store Equipment Properly

Each piece of equipment in the weight training area should be stored in a special location. People can trip or slip on those barbells, dumbbells, and weight plates left unattended or those not placed in their proper locations. Make sure you place your equipment in the appropriate locations; this applies to your equipment at home as well as to that in a weight training facility. At home there may be an added danger if children are able to climb on equipment or to try to lift plates and bars that are too heavy for them. Secure weight training equipment so that children do not have access to it without your supervision.

Using Machines

Although the mechanics of lifting on a machine are less complicated, following a few steps will help ensure safe lifting:

- Always select an appropriate load and insert selector keys all the way in.
- Adjust levers and seats to accommodate your body size, and refer to adjustment illustrations (if provided). If illustrations do not exist or you are not sure how to make adjustments, request help from a qualified person.
- Establish a stable support base when performing exercises that involve positioning your feet on the floor or positioning your head, torso, hips, or legs on or against the equipment.
- Assume a stable position on seats or rollers.
- Fasten seat belts securely (if provided).
- Perform exercises through the full range of motion and always in a slow and controlled manner.
- Do not allow the weight stack to bounce during the lowering phases or to hit the pulleys during the raising phases.

If equipment doesn't work properly, ask for help. Never place your hands or fingers between weight stacks to dislodge a selector key that sticks, and keep your hands and fingers away from the chains, belts, pulleys, and cams.

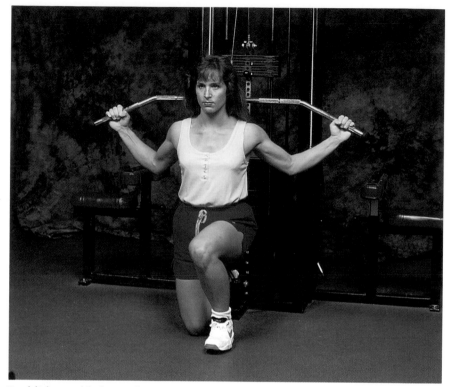

Establish a stable base of support when working on machines.

5

Warming Up and Cooling Down

The warm-up is an essential part of any well-conceived weight training program. Warm-up activities raise the body temperature and increase blood flow to the muscles, making them more pliable and less likely to become injured when challenged to perform against heavy loads. Activities such as walking, jogging, stationary cycling, stair climbing/ stepping, rowing, and rope skipping are excellent general body warm-up exercises. Another type of warm-up involves actually performing the exercise that you are warming up for but with a very light load for 8 to 15 repetitions. This specific (versus general) type of warm-up provides the opportunity for you to get your brain and muscles working in harmony before they are taxed with heavier loads. It also gives you the chance to acquire a better sense or "feel" for which muscles are involved and how to get them more involved in the exercise. Once you have completed 10 or 15 minutes of general warm-up, consider performing 8 to 15 repetitions before the first set of each exercise. The combination of both types of warm-up will prepare you mentally as well as physically for the training session.

Stretching

You should include stretching activities for each major muscle group and several for the lower back at the end of the warm-up period. Stretching after the warm-up is more successful than before it, because muscles are more flexible and more easily stretched at this time. Be careful when executing stretching exercises; otherwise, you may injure yourself. Follow these guidelines as you stretch:

- Move slowly into the stretch position, stretching to a point where you can feel tension, not pain!
- Relax, breathe in deeply, then exhale.
- Hold the stretch for 10 seconds, then return slowly to the original position.
- Perform each stretch at least twice.

Chest and Shoulders

Grasp your hands together behind your back and slowly lift your arms upward. If you are not able to grasp your hands, simply reach back as far as possible. For an additional stretch, bend at the waist and raise your arms higher.

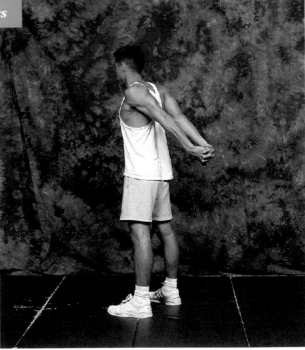

Upper Back, Shoulders, and Arms

With your right hand, grasp your left elbow and pull it slowly across your chest toward your right shoulder. You will feel the stretch along the outside of your left shoulder and arm. Repeat with the other arm.

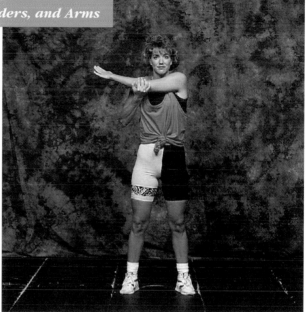

Shoulders and Triceps

Bring both arms over head and hold your left elbow with your right hand. Bend your left arm at the elbow, and let your left hand rest against right shoulder. Pull with your right hand to slowly move the left elbow behind your head until you feel a stretch. Repeat with the other arm.

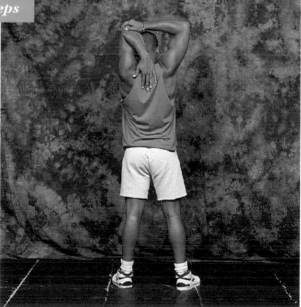

Back and Hips

Sit with your legs straight in front of you. Bend your right leg, cross it over your left knee, and place the sole of your right foot flat on the floor. Next, push against the outside of your upper right thigh with your left elbow, just above the knee. Place your right hand behind you, then

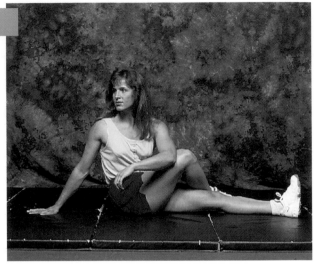

slowly rotate your upper body toward your right hand and arm. You should feel the stretch in your upper and lower back, hips, and buttocks.

Quadriceps

Using a wall or stationary object for balance, grasp your right foot with the left hand and pull so that your heel moves toward your right buttock (the alignment of foot and buttock is important to avoid stress on the knee). You should feel the stretch along the front of your right thigh. Repeat with the other leg.

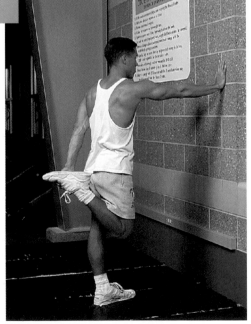

Hamstrings and Lower Back

Sit with your legs straight in front of you. Flex your right leg so that it lightly touches the inside of your left knee. Slowly bend forward from the hips toward your left foot until you feel tension in the back of your left thigh. Be sure to keep the toes of your left foot pointing up while your ankles and toes are relaxed. Repeat on the opposite side.

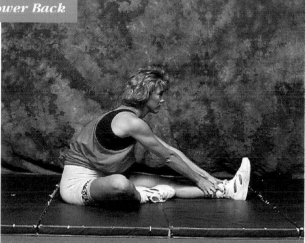

Calves

Stand about 2 feet away from a wall or stationary object. With your feet slightly apart and your knees locked, lean forward. Keep your heels on the floor and your back straight. As your hips move toward the wall, you will feel the stretch in your calves.

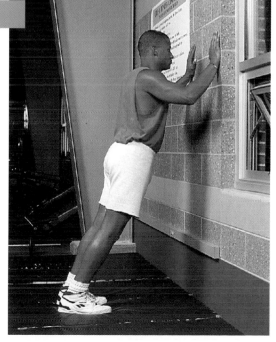

Cooling Down

Stopping abruptly when you finish your last set of exercises may cause you to become dizzy and/or nauseated. Cooling down with a 5- to 10-minute walk, an easy jog, or a series of stretching exercises will provide time to recirculate blood back to the heart from specific muscle groups, which will help avoid such problems as dizziness or nausea. Stretching during the cool-down period also provides an ideal opportunity to improve your flexibility, because the muscles and connective tissue surrounding the joints are warmer during the cool-down period than at any other time in the training session. An additional benefit of stretching during the cool-down is that it may speed your recovery from muscle soreness.

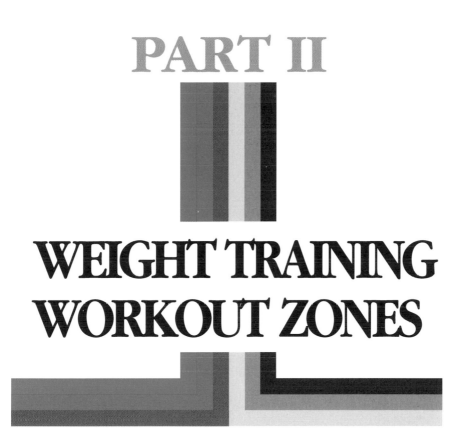

PART II

WEIGHT TRAINING WORKOUT ZONES

Part II is organized into six color-coded workout zones. Each workout is placed in a zone according to its intensity. Green workouts are the easiest and take the least time to complete, followed by the Blue, Purple, Yellow, and Orange workouts. Red workouts are the hardest and take the greatest amount of time to complete. Within each of the zones, you'll have an opportunity to select workouts that are designed to produce *muscle toning, body shaping,* or *strength development* outcomes. Which outcome is best suited to your goals and training status?

Setting Your Goals

Setting goals encourages you to make a commitment to training, which in turn motivates you to work out harder. To develop helpful goals, you need to determine both your current fitness level and what you want from weight training.

Take a few minutes now to consider your goals and what you want out of weight training. (You may want to review chapter 1 for a more detailed explanation of the terms muscle toning, body shaping, and strength training and how they relate to your weight training goals.) Are you looking to tone and define your muscles without large increases in muscle size? If so, then the muscle toning workouts are probably best for you.

Do you want to firm muscles and increase muscle definition as well as increase size? If losing fat from certain areas while increasing the size of some muscles is your goal, then the body shaping workouts are the ones to choose.

Do you seek improvement in strength for occupational, recreational, or everyday tasks or competitive sports activities? If so, follow the strength training workouts.

After you have identified your goals for weight training, write them down. Check back periodically to assess your progress, and reassess your goals as needed.

Choosing Your First Training Zone

The goals you listed identify the type of training outcome you want. Now, you need to determine which workout zone matches your current weight training fitness level by referring back to your score on the weight training fitness test (see chapter 3).

Now, look at the table on page 43. Use both your past weight training experience and the results of the bench press test to select the appropriate workout zone. For example, if you are new to weight training, have done some weight training in the past but not recently, or if you scored in the "low" fitness classification on the bench press test, start with the workouts in the Green zone. If you have been training recently but scored in the "low" fitness classification, start in the Blue zone.

Remember that the bench press test is only a guideline. If you are older than 35 or younger than 15 and have not been weight training on a regular basis, you should start in the Green or Blue zone regardless of how you scored on the test. If you feel that the workouts in your starting zone are too difficult, move to an easier one.

Weight Training Fitness Levels and Corresponding Workout Zone Categories		
Weight training fitness level	Starting zone for untrained	Starting zone for trained
Low	Green	Blue
Average	Purple	Yellow
High	Orange	Red

Understanding the Workout Zones

In each zone, the workouts are separated by the desired training outcome. Each workout provides the following information:

- The total time it will take to complete the workout, including warm-up and cool-down periods.
- The number of weeks and the number of times per week you will complete the workout—for example, you should perform Green Workout 1 over the course of 2 weeks at a rate of two nonconsecutive training sessions per week.
- A description of the weight training session in detail, including the exercises you are to perform, the number of reps and sets, and the muscle groups worked. Note that free weight exercises are to be performed with a barbell unless the exercise is specifically called a dumbbell exercise.
- Guidelines for the duration and type of warm-up and cool-down exercises you should perform.
- A recommendation for how much time you should spend between sets and exercises. During this time period, relax by simply sitting or standing at your exercise station, lightly stretching the muscles you have just exercised, or preparing the bar, dumbbell, or machine for your next set or exercise.
- An estimate of the number of calories you'll burn while completing the workout.
- Workout tips to answer common concerns or questions you may have.

Once you have completed the workouts in each zone, you have the option to repeat the zone, continue to the next zone, or design your own more personalized program. If you are curious about your progress, you can reassess yourself in the bench press test described in chapter 3. Whatever path you choose, be sure to follow the guidelines in chapter 4 to ensure your continued success. Good luck!

Green Zone

The Green zone is for you if you are new to weight training or if you have not been weight training recently and scored in the "Low" fitness classification in chapter 3. The very-low-intensity workouts in this zone are structured to gradually initiate you to weight training and to make you feel more confident and comfortable in the weight room.

Zone Highlights

The Green zone uses four 1-week training periods for each training outcome. There is one exercise for each of the seven major muscle groups: chest, back, shoulders, front of the upper arm (biceps), back of the upper arm (triceps), thighs, and abdomen. If there are any exercises you have never performed or if you are unsure about the correct exercise techniques, please refer to Appendix A or consult a professional. Remember to use a spotter in all free weight exercises that require one.

- The **muscle toning** program includes 2 days of training a week; the **body shaping** and **strength training** programs include 3 days.
- The number of sets increases from one to two in the third week of all three programs.

Choosing Your Training Days

It is important not to weight train the same muscles on 2 consecutive days or, on the other hand, to allow more than 3 days to go by between workouts. In either case you would be compromising your improvements. So, for example, for the muscle toning program you might follow a Monday/Thursday, Tuesday/Friday, or Wednesday/Saturday regime. The body shaping and strength training workouts could be performed on a Monday/Wednesday/Friday or a Tuesday/Thursday/Saturday schedule.

MUSCLE TONING

TOTAL TIME: 47 minutes

WEEKS: 1 and 2
DAYS OF THE WEEK: 2 nonconsecutive days
WARM-UP: Easy jogging or rope skipping for 5 minutes, then stretching

EXERCISES: 17 minutes

#	Muscle group	Reps	Sets	Free weight	Pivot machine	Cam machine
1	Chest	12-15	1	Bench press	Bench press	Chest press
2	Back	12-15	1	Bent over row	Seated row	Rowing exercise
3	Shoulder	12-15	1	Standing press	Seated press	Shoulder press
4	Front of arm	12-15	1	Biceps curl	Low pulley curl	Preacher curl
5	Back of arm	12-15	1	Dumbbell triceps extension	Triceps push-down	Triceps extension
6	Thigh	12-15	1	Lunge	Leg press	Dual leg press
7	Abdomen	12-15	1	Trunk curl	Trunk curl	Trunk curl

REST PERIOD: 30 seconds
COOL-DOWN: Slow walking for 5 minutes, then stretching
APPROXIMATE CALORIES EXPENDED: 160-190

WORKOUT TIPS

You may want to rest for up to 60 seconds between sets/exercises for your first or second week of training, or both.

2 W O R K O U T

TOTAL TIME: 54 minutes

WEEKS: 3 and 4
DAYS OF THE WEEK: 2 nonconsecutive days
WARM-UP: Easy jogging or rope skipping for 5 minutes, then stretching

EXERCISES: 24 minutes

#	Muscle group	Reps	Sets	Free weight	Pivot machine	Cam machine
1	Chest	12-15	2	Bench press	Bench press	Chest press
2	Back	12-15	2	Bent over row	Seated row	Rowing exercise
3	Shoulder	12-15	2	Standing press	Seated press	Shoulder press
4	Front of arm	12-15	2	Biceps curl	Low pulley curl	Preacher curl
5	Back of arm	12-15	2	Dumbbell triceps extension	Triceps push-down	Triceps extension
6	Thigh	12-15	2	Lunge	Leg press	Dual leg press
7	Abdomen	12-15	2	Trunk curl	Trunk curl	Trunk curl

REST PERIOD: 30 seconds
COOL-DOWN: Slow walking for 5 minutes, then stretching
APPROXIMATE CALORIES EXPENDED: 190-220

WORKOUT TIPS

If you are having difficulty adjusting to performing two sets, you can complete one set of each exercise and then start over and perform the second set of each exercise (as opposed to doing two sets of each exercise back-to-back).

BODY SHAPING

TOTAL TIME: 47 minutes

WEEKS: 1 and 2
DAYS OF THE WEEK: 3 nonconsecutive days
WARM-UP: Easy jogging or rope skipping for 5 minutes, then stretching

EXERCISES: 17 minutes

#	Muscle group	Reps	Sets	Free weight	Pivot machine	Cam machine
1	Chest	12-15	1	Bench press	Bench press	Chest press
2	Back	12-15	1	Bent over row	Seated row	Rowing exercise
3	Shoulder	12-15	1	Standing press	Seated press	Shoulder press
4	Front of arm	12-15	1	Biceps curl	Low pulley curl	Preacher curl
5	Back of arm	12-15	1	Dumbbell triceps extension	Triceps push-down	Triceps extension
6	Thigh	12-15	1	Lunge	Leg press	Dual leg press
7	Abdomen	12-15	1	Trunk curl	Trunk curl	Trunk curl

REST PERIOD: 30 seconds
COOL-DOWN: Slow walking for 5 minutes, then stretching
APPROXIMATE CALORIES EXPENDED: 160-190

WORKOUT TIPS

You may want to rest for up to 60 seconds between sets/exercises for your first or second week of training, or both.

2 WORKOUT

TOTAL TIME: 54 minutes

WEEKS: 3 and 4
DAYS OF THE WEEK: 3 nonconsecutive days
WARM-UP: Easy jogging or rope skipping for 5 minutes, then stretching

EXERCISES: 24 minutes

#	Muscle group	Reps	Sets	Free weight	Pivot machine	Cam machine
1	Chest	12-15	2	Bench press	Bench press	Chest press
2	Back	12-15	2	Bent over row	Seated row	Rowing exercise
3	Shoulder	12-15	2	Standing press	Seated press	Shoulder press
4	Front of arm	12-15	2	Biceps curl	Low pulley curl	Preacher curl
5	Back of arm	12-15	2	Dumbbell triceps extension	Triceps push-down	Triceps extension
6	Thigh	12-15	2	Lunge	Leg press	Dual leg press
7	Abdomen	12-15	2	Trunk curl	Trunk curl	Trunk curl

REST PERIOD: 30 seconds
COOL-DOWN: Slow walking for 5 minutes, then stretching
APPROXIMATE CALORIES EXPENDED: 190-220

WORKOUT TIPS

If you are having difficulty adjusting to performing two sets, you can complete one set of each exercise and then start over and perform the second set of each exercise (as opposed to doing two sets of each exercise back-to-back).

STRENGTH TRAINING

TOTAL TIME: 47 minutes

WEEKS: 1 and 2
DAYS OF THE WEEK: 3 nonconsecutive days
WARM-UP: Easy jogging or rope skipping for 5 minutes,
then stretching

EXERCISES: 17 minutes

#	Muscle group	Reps	Sets	Free weight	Pivot machine	Cam machine
1	Chest	12-15	1	Bench press	Bench press	Chest press
2	Back	12-15	1	Bent over row	Seated row	Rowing exercise
3	Shoulder	12-15	1	Standing press	Seated press	Shoulder press
4	Front of arm	12-15	1	Biceps curl	Low pulley curl	Preacher curl
5	Back of arm	12-15	1	Dumbbell triceps extension	Triceps push-down	Triceps extension
6	Thigh	12-15	1	Lunge	Leg press	Dual leg press
7	Abdomen	12-15	1	Trunk curl	Trunk curl	Trunk curl

REST PERIOD: 30 seconds
COOL-DOWN: Slow walking for 5 minutes, then stretching
APPROXIMATE CALORIES EXPENDED: 160-190

WORKOUT TIPS

You may want to rest for up to 60 seconds between sets/exercises
for your first or second week of training, or both.

STRENGTH TRAINING

TOTAL TIME: 54 minutes

WEEKS: 3 and 4
DAYS OF THE WEEK: 3 nonconsecutive days
WARM-UP: Easy jogging or rope skipping for 5 minutes, then stretching

EXERCISES: 24 minutes

#	Muscle group	Reps	Sets	Free weight	Pivot machine	Cam machine
1	Chest	12-15	2	Bench press	Bench press	Chest press
2	Back	12-15	2	Bent over row	Seated row	Rowing exercise
3	Shoulder	12-15	2	Standing press	Seated press	Shoulder press
4	Front of arm	12-15	2	Biceps curl	Low pulley curl	Preacher curl
5	Back of arm	12-15	2	Dumbbell triceps extension	Triceps push-down	Triceps extension
6	Thigh	12-15	2	Lunge	Leg press	Dual leg press
7	Abdomen	12-15	2	Trunk curl	Trunk curl	Trunk curl

REST PERIOD: 30 seconds
COOL-DOWN: Slow walking for 5 minutes, then stretching
APPROXIMATE CALORIES EXPENDED: 190-220

WORKOUT TIPS

If you are having difficulty adjusting to performing two sets, you can complete one set of each exercise and then start over and perform the second set of each exercise (as opposed to doing two sets of each exercise back-to-back).

7

Blue Zone

The Blue zone is for you if you have been weight training recently on a consistent basis but scored in the "Low" fitness classification in chapter 3 or if you completed the Green zone and are looking for a more advanced program. The workouts in this zone provide a solid base for the more intense zones to follow.

Zone Highlights

The Blue zone uses four 1-week training periods for each training outcome. There is one exercise for each of the seven major muscle groups: chest, back, shoulders, front of the upper arm (biceps), back of the upper arm (triceps), thighs, and abdomen. If there are any exercises you have never performed or if you are unsure about the correct exercise techniques, please review Appendix A or consult a professional. Remember to use a spotter in all free weight exercises that require one.

- The **muscle toning** program continues the 12 to 15 reps from the Green zone and adds another set (now you will be doing three) during the two weekly workouts.
- The **body shaping** program gradually decreases the number of reps to 10 to 12 but retains three sessions a week. Remember, as the number of reps decreases, you should increase the loads (chapter 12 can assist you in this process).

- The **strength training** program gradually decreases the number of reps to 8 to 10 but still retains three sessions a week. Remember, as the number of reps decreases, you should increase the loads.

Choosing Your Training Days

As in the Green zone, the suggested training days for the muscle toning program are either a Monday/Thursday, Tuesday/Friday, or Wednesday/Saturday regime. The body shaping and the strength training workouts could be performed on a Monday/Wednesday/Friday or a Tuesday/Thursday/Saturday schedule.

MUSCLE TONING

TOTAL TIME: 58 minutes

WEEKS: 1 and 2
DAYS OF THE WEEK: 2 nonconsecutive days
WARM-UP: Easy jogging or rope skipping for 5 minutes, then stretching

EXERCISES: 28 minutes

#	Muscle group	Reps	Sets	Free weight	Pivot machine	Cam machine
1	Chest	12-15	3	Bench press	Bench press	Chest press
2	Back	12-15	2	Bent over row	Seated row	Rowing exercise
3	Shoulder	12-15	3	Standing press	Seated press	Shoulder press
4	Front of arm	12-15	2	Biceps curl	Low pulley curl	Preacher curl
5	Back of arm	12-15	2	Dumbbell triceps extension	Triceps push-down	Triceps extension
6	Thigh	12-15	3	Lunge	Leg press	Dual leg press
7	Abdomen	12-15	2	Trunk curl	Trunk curl	Trunk curl

REST PERIOD: 30 seconds
COOL-DOWN: Slow walking for 5 minutes, then stretching
APPROXIMATE CALORIES EXPENDED: 210-240

WORKOUT TIPS

At this point, you should be able to perform the required two or three sets back-to-back.

MUSCLE TONING

2 WORKOUT

TOTAL TIME: 1 hour, 1 minute

WEEKS: 3 and 4
DAYS OF THE WEEK: 2 nonconsecutive days
WARM-UP: Easy jogging or rope skipping for 5 minutes, then stretching

EXERCISES: 31 minutes

#	Muscle group	Reps	Sets	Free weight	Pivot machine	Cam machine
1	Chest	12-15	3	Bench press	Bench press	Chest press
2	Back	12-15	3	Bent over row	Seated row	Rowing exercise
3	Shoulder	12-15	3	Standing press	Seated press	Shoulder press
4	Front of arm	12-15	3	Biceps curl	Low pulley curl	Preacher curl
5	Back of arm	12-15	3	Dumbbell triceps extension	Triceps push-down	Triceps extension
6	Thigh	12-15	3	Lunge	Leg press	Dual leg press
7	Abdomen	12-15	3	Trunk curl	Trunk curl	Trunk curl

REST PERIOD: 30 seconds
COOL-DOWN: Slow walking for 5 minutes, then stretching
APPROXIMATE CALORIES EXPENDED: 225-255

WORKOUT TIPS

Challenge yourself to perform 17 repetitions per set in exercises 1 through 6. If you are successful, use the 2-for-2 rule described in chapter 12 to help you make load increases.

BODY SHAPING

TOTAL TIME: 1 hour, 1 minute

WEEKS: 1 and 2
DAYS OF THE WEEK: 3 nonconsecutive days
WARM-UP: Easy jogging or rope skipping for 5 minutes, then stretching

EXERCISES: 31 minutes

#	Muscle group	Reps	Sets	Free weight	Pivot machine	Cam machine
1	Chest	10-12	2	Bench press	Bench press	Chest press
2	Back	12-15	2	Bent over row	Seated row	Rowing exercise
3	Shoulder	10-12	2	Standing press	Seated press	Shoulder press
4	Front of arm	12-15	2	Biceps curl	Low pulley curl	Preacher curl
5	Back of arm	12-15	2	Dumbbell triceps extension	Triceps push-down	Triceps extension
6	Thigh	10-12	2	Lunge	Leg press	Dual leg press
7	Abdomen	15-25	2	Trunk curl	Trunk curl	Trunk curl

REST PERIOD: 1 minute
COOL-DOWN: Slow walking for 5 minutes, then stretching
APPROXIMATE CALORIES EXPENDED: 225-255

WORKOUT TIPS

When you make the change to performing sets of 10 to 12 reps from the 12 to 15 reps used in the Green zone, a general guideline is to add 5 to 10 pounds to your upper body exercises and 10 to 20 pounds to your lower body exercises. Consult chapter 12 for a more specific method of determining new loads. At this point, you should be able to perform the required two or three sets back-to-back. Note that you are now doing sets of 15 to 25 reps for your abdominal exercise.

BODY SHAPING

2 W O R K O U T

TOTAL TIME: 1 hour, 1 minute

WEEKS: 3 and 4
DAYS OF THE WEEK: 3 nonconsecutive days
WARM-UP: Easy jogging or rope skipping for 5 minutes, then stretching

EXERCISES: 31 minutes

#	Muscle group	Reps	Sets	Free weight	Pivot machine	Cam machine
1	Chest	10-12	2	Bench press	Bench press	Chest press
2	Back	10-12	2	Bent over row	Seated row	Rowing exercise
3	Shoulder	10-12	2	Standing press	Seated press	Shoulder press
4	Front of arm	10-12	2	Biceps curl	Low pulley curl	Preacher curl
5	Back of arm	10-12	2	Dumbbell triceps extension	Triceps push-down	Triceps extension
6	Thigh	10-12	2	Lunge	Leg press	Dual leg press
7	Abdomen	15-25	2	Trunk curl	Trunk curl	Trunk curl

REST PERIOD: 1 minute
COOL-DOWN: Slow walking for 5 minutes, then stretching
APPROXIMATE CALORIES EXPENDED: 225-255

WORKOUT TIPS

Challenge yourself to perform 14 repetitions per set in exercises 1 through 6. If you are successful, use the 2-for-2 rule described in chapter 12 to help you make load increases.

STRENGTH TRAINING

TOTAL TIME: 1 hour, 1 minute

WEEKS: 1 and 2
DAYS OF THE WEEK: 3 nonconsecutive days
WARM-UP: Easy jogging or rope skipping for 5 minutes, then stretching

EXERCISES: 31 minutes

#	Muscle group	Reps	Sets	Free weight	Pivot machine	Cam machine
1	Chest	8-10	2	Bench press	Bench press	Chest press
2	Back	12-15	2	Bent over row	Seated row	Rowing exercise
3	Shoulder	8-10	2	Standing press	Seated press	Shoulder press
4	Front of arm	12-15	2	Biceps curl	Low pulley curl	Preacher curl
5	Back of arm	12-15	2	Dumbbell triceps extension	Triceps push-down	Triceps extension
6	Thigh	8-10	2	Lunge	Leg press	Dual leg press
7	Abdomen	15-25	2	Trunk curl	Trunk curl	Trunk curl

REST PERIOD: 1 minute
COOL-DOWN: Slow walking for 5 minutes, then stretching
APPROXIMATE CALORIES EXPENDED: 225-255

WORKOUT TIPS

When you make the change to performing sets of 8 to 10 reps from the 12 to 15 reps used in the Green zone, a general guideline is to add 10 to 20 pounds to your upper body exercises and 15 to 25 pounds to your lower body exercises. Consult chapter 12 for a more specific method of determining new loads. At this point, you should be able to perform the required two sets back-to-back. Note that you are now doing sets of 15 to 25 reps for your abdominal exercise.

2 W O R K O U T

TOTAL TIME: 1 hour, 1 minute

WEEKS: 3 and 4
DAYS OF THE WEEK: 3 nonconsecutive days
WARM-UP: Easy jogging or rope skipping for 5 minutes, then stretching

EXERCISES: 31 minutes

#	Muscle group	Reps	Sets	Free weight	Pivot machine	Cam machine
1	Chest	8-10	2	Bench press	Bench press	Chest press
2	Back	8-10	2	Bent over row	Seated row	Rowing exercise
3	Shoulder	8-10	2	Standing press	Seated press	Shoulder press
4	Front of arm	8-10	2	Biceps curl	Low pulley curl	Preacher curl
5	Back of arm	8-10	2	Dumbbell triceps extension	Triceps push-down	Triceps extension
6	Thigh	8-10	2	Lunge	Leg press	Dual leg press
7	Abdomen	15-25	2	Trunk curl	Trunk curl	Trunk curl

REST PERIOD: 1 minute
COOL-DOWN: Slow walking for 5 minutes, then stretching
APPROXIMATE CALORIES EXPENDED: 225-255

WORKOUT TIPS

Challenge yourself to perform 12 repetitions per set in exercises 1 through 6. If you are successful, use the 2-for-2 rule to help you make load increases.

8

Purple Zone

The Purple zone is for you if you have not been weight training recently on a consistent basis and scored in the "Average" fitness classification in chapter 3 or if you completed the Blue zone and are looking for a more advanced program. The workouts in this zone are more intense, and they help provide a base for the workouts in the advanced zones.

Zone Highlights

The Purple zone uses four 1-week training periods for each training outcome. If there are any exercises you have never performed or if you are unsure about the correct exercise techniques, please refer to Appendix A or consult a professional. Remember to use a spotter for free weight exercises that require one.

- The **muscle toning** program includes seven exercises using 12 to 15 reps per set. There is an exercise for each of the seven major muscle groups: chest, back, shoulders, biceps, triceps, thighs, and abdomen. A major change in this zone is that you will be completing three workouts a week instead of two. Because of this increase, weeks 1 and 2 require you only to complete two sets per exercise. Weeks 3 and 4 gradually return you to three sets.
- The **body shaping** program involves the same exercises as the muscle toning program, but you should perform 10 to 12 reps for three sets by the third week of the workouts.

- The **strength training** program consists of four workouts each week; your program is divided into 2 upper body and 2 lower body training days. Because of the increase in the number of weekly workouts, you will be performing only one to two sets of 8 to 10 reps in seven upper body and six lower body exercises. The upper body exercises include two each for the chest and back and one for the shoulders, biceps, and the triceps. The lower body exercises include two for the thighs and one for the back of the thigh (hamstrings), the front of the thigh (quadriceps), the calves, and the abdomen.

Choosing Your Training Days

It is important not to weight train the same muscle group on 2 consecutive days or, on the other hand, to allow more than 3 days to go by between sessions. In either case you would be compromising the benefits you receive from working out. So, for the muscle toning and body shaping workouts you might follow a Monday/Wednesday/Friday or a Tuesday/Thursday/Saturday schedule.

To determine the most effective way to complete four strength training sessions per week, simply choose from the following table one of the three options for your training days. It is best to choose an option that you can adhere to consistently and one that is convenient for you. Each option provides two workouts each for your upper and lower body and spreads out all of the workouts so that you have sufficient rest days between similar weight training sessions.

Training day option	Upper body workouts	Lower body workouts
1	Mondays and Thursdays	Tuesdays and Fridays
2	Sundays and Wednesdays	Mondays and Thursdays
3	Tuesdays and Fridays	Wednesdays and Saturdays

MUSCLE TONING

TOTAL TIME: 54 minutes

WEEKS: 1 and 2
DAYS OF THE WEEK: 3 nonconsecutive days
WARM-UP: Easy jogging or rope skipping for 5 minutes, then stretching

EXERCISES: 24 minutes

#	Muscle group	Reps	Sets	Free weight	Pivot machine	Cam machine
1	Chest	12-15	2	Bench press	Bench press	Chest press
2	Back	12-15	2	Bent over row	Seated row	Rowing exercise
3	Shoulder	12-15	2	Standing press	Seated press	Shoulder press
4	Front of arm	12-15	2	Biceps curl	Low pulley curl	Preacher curl
5	Back of arm	12-15	2	Dumbbell triceps extension	Triceps push-down	Triceps extension
6	Thigh	12-15	2	Lunge	Leg press	Dual leg press
7	Abdomen	15-25	2	Trunk curl	Trunk curl	Trunk curl

REST PERIOD: 30 seconds
COOL-DOWN: Slow walking for 5 minutes, then stretching
APPROXIMATE CALORIES EXPENDED: 230-260

WORKOUT TIPS

Be sure to spread out your weight training sessions throughout the week; you need at least 1 rest day (but no more than 3) between workouts. A common program is Monday/Wednesday/Friday or Tuesday/Thursday/one weekend day. Note that you are now doing sets of 15 to 25 reps for your abdominal exercise.

MUSCLE TONING

TOTAL TIME: 58 minutes

WEEKS: 3 and 4
DAYS OF THE WEEK: 3 nonconsecutive days
WARM-UP: Easy jogging or rope skipping for 5 minutes,
   then stretching

EXERCISES: 28 minutes

#	Muscle group	Reps	Sets	Free weight	Pivot machine	Cam machine
1	Chest	12-15	3	Bench press	Bench press	Chest press
2	Back	12-15	2	Bent over row	Seated row	Rowing exercise
3	Shoulder	12-15	3	Standing press	Seated press	Shoulder press
4	Front of arm	12-15	2	Biceps curl	Low pulley curl	Preacher curl
5	Back of arm	12-15	2	Dumbbell triceps extension	Triceps push-down	Triceps extension
6	Thigh	12-15	3	Lunge	Leg press	Dual leg press
7	Abdomen	15-25	3	Trunk curl	Trunk curl	Trunk curl

REST PERIOD: 30 seconds
COOL-DOWN: Slow walking for 5 minutes, then stretching
APPROXIMATE CALORIES EXPENDED: 260-290

WORKOUT TIPS

If you feel that performing three back-to-back sets is too difficult,
complete two back-to-back sets in all of the exercises first and then
complete a third set for exercises 1, 3, 6, and 7 only.

BODY SHAPING

TOTAL TIME: 1 hour, 6 minutes

WEEKS: 1 and 2
DAYS OF THE WEEK: 3 nonconsecutive days
WARM-UP: Easy jogging or rope skipping for 5 minutes, then stretching

EXERCISES: 36 minutes

#	Muscle group	Reps	Sets	Free weight	Pivot machine	Cam machine
1	Chest	10-12	3	Bench press	Bench press	Chest press
2	Back	10-12	2	Bent over row	Seated row	Rowing exercise
3	Shoulder	10-12	3	Standing press	Seated press	Shoulder press
4	Front of arm	10-12	2	Biceps curl	Low pulley curl	Preacher curl
5	Back of arm	10-12	2	Dumbbell triceps extension	Triceps push-down	Triceps extension
6	Thigh	10-12	3	Lunge	Leg press	Dual leg press
7	Abdomen	15-25	2	Trunk curl	Trunk curl	Trunk curl

REST PERIOD: 1 minute
COOL-DOWN: Slow walking for 5 minutes, then stretching
APPROXIMATE CALORIES EXPENDED: 315-345

WORKOUT TIPS

Remember to use a spotter in the free weight version of exercises 1, 3, and 6.

BODY SHAPING

2 WORKOUT

TOTAL TIME: 1 hour, 12 minutes

WEEKS: 3 and 4
DAYS OF THE WEEK: 3 nonconsecutive days
WARM-UP: Easy jogging or rope skipping for 5 minutes, then stretching

EXERCISES: 42 minutes

#	Muscle group	Reps	Sets	Free weight	Pivot machine	Cam machine
1	Chest	10-12	3	Bench press	Bench press	Chest press
2	Back	10-12	3	Bent over row	Seated row	Rowing exercise
3	Shoulder	10-12	3	Standing press	Seated press	Shoulder press
4	Front of arm	10-12	3	Biceps curl	Low pulley curl	Preacher curl
5	Back of arm	10-12	3	Dumbbell triceps extension	Triceps push-down	Triceps extension
6	Thigh	10-12	3	Lunge	Leg press	Dual leg press
7	Abdomen	15-25	3	Trunk curl	Trunk curl	Trunk curl

REST PERIOD: 1 minute
COOL-DOWN: Slow walking for 5 minutes, then stretching
APPROXIMATE CALORIES EXPENDED: 360-390

WORKOUT TIPS

If you feel that performing three back-to-back sets is too difficult, complete two back-to-back sets of all the exercises first and then go back and complete the third set.

STRENGTH TRAINING

TOTAL TIME: 58 minutes

WEEKS: 1 and 2
DAYS OF THE WEEK: 2 nonconsecutive days
WARM-UP: Easy jogging or rope skipping for 5 minutes, then stretching

UPPER BODY EXERCISES: 28 minutes

#	Muscle group	Reps	Sets	Free weight	Pivot machine	Cam machine
1	Chest	8-10	2	Bench press	Bench press	Chest press
2	Chest	8-10	1	Dumbbell fly	Pec deck (butterfly)	Bent-arm fly
3	Back	8-10	2	Bent over row	Seated row	Rowing exercise
4	Shoulder	8-10	2	Standing press	Seated press	Shoulder press
5	Back	8-10	1	Dumbbell row	Lat pull-down	Pull-down/ pull-over exercise
6	Back of arm	8-10	2	Dumbbell triceps extension	Triceps push-down	Triceps extension
7	Front of arm	8-10	2	Biceps curl	Low pulley curl	Preacher curl

REST PERIOD: 1 minute
COOL-DOWN: Slow walking for 5 minutes, then stretching
APPROXIMATE CALORIES EXPENDED: 260-390

WORKOUT TIPS

When you make the change to four workouts per week, you will perform upper body and lower body workouts separately. This means you will have an opportunity to add new exercises and still complete your workouts in about the same amount of time. Refer to chapter 12 to determine your starting loads for new exercises.

STRENGTH TRAINING

2 WORKOUT

TOTAL TIME: 52 minutes

WEEKS: 1 and 2
DAYS OF THE WEEK: 2 nonconsecutive days
WARM-UP: Easy jogging or rope skipping for 5 minutes,
    then stretching

LOWER BODY EXERCISES: 22 minutes

#	Muscle group	Reps	Sets	Free weight	Pivot machine	Cam machine
1	Thigh	8-10	1	Squat	Leg press	Dual leg press
2	Thigh	8-10	2	Lunge	Horizontal leg press	Horizontal leg press
3	Back of thigh	8-10	1	Leg curl	Leg curl	Leg curl
4	Front of thigh	8-10	1	Leg extension	Leg extension	Leg extension
5	Calf	8-10	1	Standing calf raise	Heel raise	Heel raise
6	Abdomen	15-25	2	Trunk curl	Trunk curl	Trunk curl

REST PERIOD: 1 minute
COOL-DOWN: Slow walking for 5 minutes, then stretching
APPROXIMATE CALORIES EXPENDED: 215-245

WORKOUT TIPS

When you make the change to four workouts per week, you will perform upper body and lower body workouts separately. This means you will have an opportunity to add new exercises and still complete your workouts in about the same amount of time.

TOTAL TIME: 1 hour, 1 minute

WEEKS: 3 and 4
DAYS OF THE WEEK: 2 nonconsecutive days
WARM UP: Easy jogging or rope skipping for 5 minutes, then stretching

UPPER BODY EXERCISES: 31 minutes

#	Muscle group	Reps	Sets	Free weight	Pivot machine	Cam machine
1	Chest	8-10	2	Bench press	Bench press	Chest press
2	Chest	8-10	2	Dumbbell fly	Pec deck (butterfly)	Bent-arm fly
3	Back	8-10	2	Bent over row	Seated row	Rowing exercise
4	Shoulder	8-10	2	Standing press	Seated press	Shoulder press
5	Back	8-10	2	Dumbbell row	Lat pull-down	Pull-down/ pull-over exercise
6	Back of arm	8-10	2	Dumbbell triceps extension	Triceps push-down	Triceps extension
7	Front of arm	8-10	2	Biceps curl	Low pulley curl	Preacher curl

REST PERIOD: 1 minute
COOL-DOWN: Slow walking for 5 minutes, then stretching
APPROXIMATE CALORIES EXPENDED: 285-315

WORKOUT TIPS

You may need to readjust the loads you are using in your new exercises to successfully complete two back-to-back sets.

4 WORKOUT

TOTAL TIME: 58 minutes

WEEKS: 3 and 4
DAYS OF THE WEEK: 2 nonconsecutive days
WARM-UP: Easy jogging or rope skipping for 5 minutes, then stretching

LOWER BODY EXERCISES: 28 minutes

#	Muscle group	Reps	Sets	Free weight	Pivot machine	Cam machine
1	Thigh	8-10	2	Squat	Leg press	Dual leg press
2	Thigh	8-10	2	Lunge	Horizontal leg press	Horizontal leg press
3	Back of thigh	8-10	2	Leg curl	Leg curl	Leg curl
4	Front of thigh	8-10	2	Leg extension	Leg extension	Leg extension
5	Calf	8-10	2	Standing calf raise	Heel raise	Heel raise
6	Abdomen	15-25	2	Trunk curl	Trunk curl	Trunk curl

REST PERIOD: 1 minute
COOL-DOWN: Slow walking for 5 minutes, then stretching
APPROXIMATE CALORIES EXPENDED: 260-290

WORKOUT TIPS

You may need to readjust the loads you are using in your new exercises to successfully complete two back-to-back sets.

9

Yellow Zone

The Yellow zone is for you if you have been weight training recently on a consistent basis and scored in the "Average" fitness classification from chapter 3 or if you completed the Purple zone and are looking for a more advanced program. The workouts in this zone will help you prepare for more intense workouts in the upcoming zones.

Zone Highlights

The Yellow zone uses four 1-week training periods for each training outcome. If there are any exercises you have never performed or if you are unsure about the correct exercise techniques, please refer to Appendix A or consult a professional. Remember to use a spotter for all free weight exercises that require one.

- The first 2 weeks of the **muscle toning** program include three sets of 12 to 15 reps in seven exercises for three workouts a week. There is one exercise for each of the seven major muscle groups: chest, back, shoulders, biceps, triceps, thighs, and abdomen. Weeks 3 and 4 include three additional exercises—one set of 12 to 15 reps each for your chest, back, and calves. To determine what loads you should use in the new exercises, follow the guidelines in chapter 12.
- The **body shaping** program includes four workouts each week; your program is divided into 2 upper body and 2 lower body training days. Because of the increase in the number of weekly workouts, you will

be performing only one to two sets of 10 to 12 reps in your seven upper and six lower body exercises. The reduced number of sets provides a gradual increase in intensity. The upper body exercises include two each for the chest and back and one each for the shoulders, front of the upper arm (biceps), and back of the upper arm (triceps). The lower body exercises include two for the thighs and one each for the back of the thigh (hamstrings), the front of the thigh (quadriceps), the calves, and the abdomen. Chapter 12 will help you determine the loads for your new exercises.

- The **strength training** program includes two upper and two lower body workouts each week for two to three sets of 8 to 10 reps in each exercise. The exercises are similar to those found in the body shaping program.

Choosing Your Training Days

It is important not to weight train the same muscle group on 2 consecutive days or, on the other hand, to allow more than 3 days to go by between sessions. In either case you would be compromising your improvements. So, for the muscle toning workouts you might follow a Monday/Wednesday/Friday or a Tuesday/Thursday/Saturday schedule.

To determine the most effective way to complete four body shaping or strength training sessions per week, simply choose from the following table, one of the three options for your training days. Choose an option that you can stick to consistently and one that is convenient for you. Each option provides two workouts each for your upper and lower body and distributes the workouts so that you have sufficient rest days between similar weight training sessions.

Training day option	Upper body workouts	Lower body workouts
1	Mondays and Thursdays	Tuesdays and Fridays
2	Sundays and Wednesdays	Mondays and Thursdays
3	Tuesdays and Fridays	Wednesdays and Saturdays

TOTAL TIME: 1 hour, 1 minute

WEEKS: 1 and 2
DAYS OF THE WEEK: 3 nonconsecutive days
WARM-UP: Easy jogging or rope skipping for 5 minutes, then stretching

EXERCISES: 31 minutes

#	Muscle group	Reps	Sets	Free weight	Pivot machine	Cam machine
1	Chest	12-15	3	Bench press	Bench press	Chest press
2	Back	12-15	3	Bent over row	Seated row	Rowing exercise
3	Shoulder	12-15	3	Standing press	Seated press	Shoulder press
4	Front of arm	12-15	3	Biceps curl	Low pulley curl	Preacher curl
5	Back of arm	12-15	3	Dumbbell triceps extension	Triceps push-down	Triceps extension
6	Thigh	12-15	3	Lunge	Leg press	Dual leg press
7	Abdomen	15-25	3	Trunk curl	Trunk curl	Trunk curl

REST PERIOD: 30 seconds
COOL-DOWN: Slow walking for 5 minutes, then stretching
APPROXIMATE CALORIES EXPENDED: 225-255

WORKOUT TIPS

Challenge yourself by slightly decreasing the rest time to 15 to 20 seconds between sets. This will increase the program's difficulty without increasing the loads. Be sure not to reduce the rest period so much that you cannot perform the required number of repetitions.

TOTAL TIME: 1 hour, 4 minutes

WEEKS: 3 and 4
DAYS OF THE WEEK: 3 nonconsecutive days
WARM-UP: Easy jogging or rope skipping for 5
minutes, then stretching

EXERCISES: 34 minutes

#	Muscle group	Reps	Sets	Free weight	Pivot machine	Cam machine
1	Chest	12-15	3	Bench press	Bench press	Chest press
2	Chest	12-15	1	Dumbbell fly	Pec deck (butterfly)	Bent-arm fly
3	Back	12-15	3	Bent over row	Seated row	Rowing exercise
4	Shoulder	12-15	3	Standing press	Seated press	Shoulder press
5	Back	12-15	1	Dumbbell row	Lat pull-down	Pull-down/ pull-over exercise
6	Back of arm	12-15	3	Dumbbell triceps extension	Triceps push-down	Triceps extension
7	Front of arm	12-15	3	Biceps curl	Low pulley curl	Preacher curl
8	Thigh	12-15	3	Lunge	Leg press	Dual leg press
9	Abdomen	15-25	3	Trunk curl	Trunk curl	Trunk curl
10	Calf	12-15	1	Standing calf raise	Heel raise	Heel raise

REST PERIOD: 30 seconds
COOL-DOWN: Slow walking for 5 minutes, then stretching
APPROXIMATE CALORIES EXPENDED: 305-335

WORKOUT TIPS

Now you are completing 10 exercises per session; to learn how to perform your new exercises, consult Appendix A. The procedure described in chapter 12 will help you determine your starting loads in these exercises.

BODY SHAPING

TOTAL TIME: 58 minutes

WEEKS: 1 and 2
DAYS OF THE WEEK: 2 nonconsecutive days
WARM-UP: Easy jogging or rope skipping for 5 minutes, then stretching

UPPER BODY EXERCISES: 28 minutes

#	Muscle group	Reps	Sets	Free weight	Pivot machine	Cam machine
1	Chest	10-12	2	Bench press	Bench press	Chest press
2	Chest	10-12	1	Dumbbell fly	Pec deck (butterfly)	Bent-arm fly
3	Back	10-12	2	Bent over row	Seated row	Rowing exercise
4	Shoulder	10-12	2	Standing press	Seated press	Shoulder press
5	Back	10 12	1	Dumbbell row	Lat pull-down	Pull-down/ pull-over exercise
6	Back of arm	10-12	2	Dumbbell triceps extension	Triceps push-down	Triceps extension
7	Front of arm	10-12	2	Biceps curl	Low pulley curl	Preacher curl

REST PERIOD: 1 minute
COOL-DOWN: Slow walking for 5 minutes, then stretching
APPROXIMATE CALORIES EXPENDED: 260-290

WORKOUT TIPS

When you make the change to four workouts per week, you will perform upper body and lower body workouts separately. This means you will have an opportunity to add new exercises and still complete your workouts in about the same amount of time. Refer to chapter 12 to determine your starting loads for new exercises.

WORKOUT 2

TOTAL TIME: 52 minutes

WEEKS: 1 and 2
DAYS OF THE WEEK: 2 nonconsecutive days
WARM-UP: Easy jogging or rope skipping for 5 minutes,
  then stretching

LOWER BODY EXERCISES: 22 minutes

#	Muscle group	Reps	Sets	Free weight	Pivot machine	Cam machine
1	Thigh	10-12	1	Squat	Leg press	Dual leg press
2	Thigh	10-12	2	Lunge	Horizontal leg press	Horizontal leg press
3	Back of thigh	10-12	1	Leg curl	Leg curl	Leg curl
4	Front of thigh	10-12	1	Leg extension	Leg extension	Leg extension
5	Calf	10-12	1	Standing calf raise	Heel raise	Heel raise
6	Abdomen	15-25	2	Trunk curl	Trunk curl	Trunk curl

REST PERIOD: 1 minute
COOL-DOWN: Slow walking for 5 minutes, then stretching
APPROXIMATE CALORIES EXPENDED: 215-245

WORKOUT TIPS

When you make the change to four workouts per week, you will
perform upper body and lower body workouts separately. This
means you will have an opportunity to add new exercises and still
complete your workouts in about the same amount of time.

BODY SHAPING

TOTAL TIME: 1 hour, 1 minute

WEEKS: 3 and 4
DAYS OF THE WEEK: 2 nonconsecutive days
WARM-UP: Easy jogging or rope skipping for 5 minutes, then stretching

UPPER BODY EXERCISES: 31 minutes

#	Muscle group	Reps	Sets	Free weight	Pivot machine	Cam machine
1	Chest	8-10	2	Bench press	Bench press	Chest press
2	Chest	8-10	2	Dumbbell fly	Pec deck (butterfly)	Bent-arm fly
3	Back	8-10	2	Bent over row	Seated row	Rowing exercise
4	Shoulder	8-10	2	Standing press	Seated press	Shoulder press
5	Back	8-10	2	Dumbbell row	Lat pull-down	Pull-down/ pull-over exercise
6	Back of arm	8-10	2	Dumbbell triceps extension	Triceps push-down	Triceps extension
7	Front of arm	8-10	2	Biceps curl	Low pulley curl	Preacher curl

REST PERIOD: 1 minute
COOL-DOWN: Slow walking for 5 minutes, then stretching
APPROXIMATE CALORIES EXPENDED: 285-315

WORKOUT TIPS

You may need to readjust the loads you are using in your new exercises to successfully complete two back to back sets.

4 W
O
R
K
O
U
T

TOTAL TIME: 58 minutes

WEEKS: 3 and 4
DAYS OF THE WEEK: 2 nonconsecutive days
WARM-UP: Easy jogging or rope skipping for 5 minutes, then stretching

LOWER BODY EXERCISES: 28 minutes

#	Muscle group	Reps	Sets	Free weight	Pivot machine	Cam machine
1	Thigh	8-10	2	Squat	Leg press	Dual leg press
2	Thigh	8-10	2	Lunge	Horizontal leg press	Horizontal leg press
3	Back of thigh	8-10	2	Leg curl	Leg curl	Leg curl
4	Front of thigh	8-10	2	Leg extension	Leg extension	Leg extension
5	Calf	8-10	2	Standing calf raise	Heel raise	Heel raise
6	Abdomen	15-25	2	Trunk curl	Trunk curl	Trunk curl

REST PERIOD: 1 minute
COOL-DOWN: Slow walking for 5 minutes, then stretching
APPROXIMATE CALORIES EXPENDED: 260-290

WORKOUT TIPS

You may need to readjust the loads you are using in your new exercises to successfully complete two back-to-back sets.

TOTAL TIME: 1 hour, 4 minutes

WEEKS: 1 and 2
DAYS OF THE WEEK: 2 nonconsecutive days
WARM-UP: Easy jogging or rope skipping for 5 minutes, then stretching

UPPER BODY EXERCISES: 34 minutes

#	Muscle group	Reps	Sets	Free weight	Pivot machine	Cam machine
1	Chest	8-10	3	Bench press	Bench press	Chest press
2	Chest	8-10	2	Dumbbell fly	Pec deck (butterfly)	Bent-arm fly
3	Back	8-10	2	Bent over row	Seated row	Rowing exercise
4	Shoulder	8-10	3	Standing press	Seated press	Shoulder press
5	Back	8-10	2	Dumbbell row	Lat pull-downs	Pull-down/ pull-over exercise
6	Back of arm	8 10	2	Dumbbell triceps extension	Triceps push-down	Triceps extension
7	Front of arm	8-10	2	Biceps curl	Low pulley curl	Preacher curl

REST PERIOD: 1 minute
COOL-DOWN: Slow walking for 5 minutes, then stretching
APPROXIMATE CALORIES EXPENDED: 305-335

WORKOUT TIPS

To increase the difficulty of the major or core exercises (1 and 4), keep readjusting the load to perform 8 reps per set instead of 10. To do this, apply the 2-for-2 rule when you reach 10 reps in the last set for two consecutive workouts.

2

TOTAL TIME: 1 hour, 3 minutes

WEEKS: 1 and 2
DAYS OF THE WEEK: 2 nonconsecutive days
WARM-UP: Easy jogging or rope skipping for 5 minutes, then stretching

LOWER BODY EXERCISES: 33 minutes

#	Muscle group	Reps	Sets	Free weight	Pivot machine	Cam machine
1	Thigh	8-10	3	Squat	Leg press	Dual leg press
2	Thigh	8-10	3	Lunge	Horizontal leg press	Horizontal leg press
3	Back of thigh	8-10	2	Leg curl	Leg curl	Leg curl
4	Front of thigh	8-10	2	Leg extension	Leg extension	Leg extension
5	Calf	8-10	2	Standing calf raise	Heel raise	Heel raise
6	Abdomen	15-25	3	Trunk curl	Trunk curl	Trunk curl

REST PERIOD: 1 minute
COOL-DOWN: Slow walking for 5 minutes, then stretching
APPROXIMATE CALORIES EXPENDED: 295-325

WORKOUT TIPS

To increase the difficulty of a major or core exercise (1), keep readjusting the load to perform 8 reps per set instead of 10. To do this, apply the 2-for-2 rule when you reach 10 reps in the last set for two consecutive workouts.

TOTAL TIME: 1 hour, 12 minutes

WEEKS: 3 and 4
DAYS OF THE WEEK: 2 nonconsecutive days
WARM-UP: Easy jogging or rope skipping for 5 minutes, then stretching

UPPER BODY EXERCISES: 42 minutes

#	Muscle group	Reps	Sets	Free weight	Pivot machine	Cam machine
1	Chest	8-10	3	Bench press	Bench press	Chest press
2	Chest	8-10	3	Dumbbell fly	Pec deck (butterfly)	Bent-arm fly
3	Back	8-10	3	Bent over row	Seated row	Rowing exercise
4	Shoulder	8-10	3	Standing press	Seated press	Shoulder press
5	Back	8-10	3	Dumbbell row	Lat pull-down	Pull-down/ pull-over exercise
6	Back of arm	8-10	3	Dumbbell triceps extension	Triceps push-down	Triceps extension
7	Front of arm	8-10	3	Biceps curl	Low pulley curl	Preacher curl

REST PERIOD: 1 minute
COOL-DOWN: Slow walking for 5 minutes, then stretching
APPROXIMATE CALORIES EXPENDED: 360-390

WORKOUT TIPS

As the loads become heavier, remember to always use a spotter, especially for the free weight version of exercises 1 and 4.

4

TOTAL TIME: 1 hour, 7 minutes

WEEKS: 3 and 4
DAYS OF THE WEEK: 2 nonconsecutive days
WARM-UP: Easy jogging or rope skipping for 5 minutes, then stretching

LOWER BODY EXERCISES: 37 minutes

#	Muscle group	Reps	Sets	Free weight	Pivot machine	Cam machine
1	Thigh	8-10	3	Squat	Leg press	Dual leg press
2	Thigh	8-10	3	Lunge	Horizontal leg press	Horizontal leg press
3	Back of thigh	8-10	3	Leg curl	Leg curl	Leg curl
4	Front of thigh	8-10	3	Leg extension	Leg extension	Leg extension
5	Calf	8-10	3	Standing calf raise	Heel raise	Heel raise
6	Abdomen	15-25	3	Trunk curl	Trunk curl	Trunk curl

REST PERIOD: 1 minute
COOL-DOWN: Slow walking for 5 minutes, then stretching
APPROXIMATE CALORIES EXPENDED: 285-315

WORKOUT TIPS

As the loads become heavier, remember to always use a spotter, especially for the free weight version of exercises 1 and 2.

10

Orange Zone

The Orange zone is for you if you have not been weight training recently on a consistent basis and scored in the "High" fitness classification from chapter 3 or if you completed the Yellow zone and are looking for a more advanced program. The workouts in this zone are very intense and require dedication if you want to be successful.

Zone Highlights

The Orange zone utilizes four 1-week training periods for each training outcome. If there are any exercises you have never performed or if you are unsure about the correct exercise techniques, please refer to Appendix A or consult a professional. Remember to use a spotter for free weight exercises that require one.

- The **muscle toning** program includes two to three sets of 12 to 15 reps in 10 exercises for three workouts a week. There is one exercise for each major muscle group (except where noted): chest (two exercises), back (two exercises), shoulders, front of the upper arm (biceps), back of the upper arm (triceps), thighs, calves, and abdomen.
- The **body shaping** program continues to add sets to the 4 training days (2 upper body and 2 lower body) weekly; you will perform two to three sets of 10 to 12 reps in each of your seven upper body and six lower body exercises. The upper body exercises include two each

for the chest and back and one each for the shoulders, the biceps, and the triceps. The lower body exercises include two for the thighs and one for the back of the thigh (hamstrings), the front of the thigh (quadriceps), the calves, and the abdomen.

- The **strength training** program includes two upper body and two lower body workouts each week using the same exercises as in the body shaping program. However, depending on the exercise, the program now has different repetition goals: 6 to 8 reps for the major or core exercises and 8 to 10 for all others. In this zone you will begin performing weight-lifting exercises as part of your warm-up. Follow the warm-up procedure outlined in the warm-up section of each strength training workout. Warm-up sets are not counted in the number of sets you are scheduled to complete. During the last 2 weeks of this zone, you will complete four sets in the core exercises.

Choosing Your Training Days

It is important not to weight train the same muscle group on 2 consecutive days or, on the other hand, to allow more than 3 days to go by between sessions. In either case you would be compromising your improvements. So, for the muscle toning workouts you might follow a Monday/Wednesday/Friday or a Tuesday/Thursday/Saturday schedule.

To determine the most effective way to complete four body shaping or strength training sessions per week, simply choose from the following table one of the three options for your training days. Choose an option that you can stick to consistently and one that is convenient for you. Each option provides two workouts each for your upper and lower body and distributes the workouts so that you have sufficient rest days between similar weight training sessions.

Training day option	Upper body workouts	Lower body workouts
1	Mondays and Thursdays	Tuesdays and Fridays
2	Sundays and Wednesdays	Mondays and Thursdays
3	Tuesdays and Fridays	Wednesdays and Saturdays

MUSCLE TONING

TOTAL TIME: 1 hour, 7 minutes

WEEKS: 1 and 2
DAYS OF THE WEEK: 3 nonconsecutive days
WARM-UP: Easy jogging or rope skipping for 5 minutes, then stretching

EXERCISES: 37 minutes

#	Muscle group	Reps	Sets	Free weight	Pivot machine	Cam machine
1	Chest	12-15	3	Bench press	Bench press	Chest press
2	Chest	12-15	2	Dumbbell fly	Pec deck (butterfly)	Bent-arm fly
3	Back	12-15	3	Bent over row	Seated row	Rowing exercise
4	Shoulder	12-15	3	Standing press	Seated press	Shoulder press
5	Back	12-15	2	Dumbbell row	Lat pull-down	Pull-down/ pull-over exercise
6	Back of arm	12-15	3	Dumbbell triceps extension	Triceps push-down	Triceps extension
7	Front of arm	12-15	3	Biceps curl	Low pulley curl	Preacher curl
8	Thigh	12-15	3	Lunge	Leg press	Dual leg press
9	Abdomen	15-25	3	Trunk curl	Trunk curl	Trunk curl
10	Calf	12-15	2	Standing calf raise	Heel raise	Heel raise

REST PERIOD: 30 seconds
COOL-DOWN: Slow walking for 5 minutes, then stretching
APPROXIMATE CALORIES EXPENDED: 375-405

WORKOUT TIPS

Be sure to perform the new exercises (2, 5, and 10) back-to-back and in the order listed above.

MUSCLE TONING

2 WORKOUT

TOTAL TIME: 1 hour, 10 minutes

WEEKS: 1 and 2
DAYS OF THE WEEK: 3 nonconsecutive days
WARM-UP: Easy jogging or rope skipping for 5 minutes, then stretching

EXERCISES: 40 minutes

#	Muscle group	Reps	Sets	Free weight	Pivot machine	Cam machine
1	Chest	12-15	3	Bench press	Bench press	Chest press
2	Chest	12-15	3	Dumbbell fly	Pec deck (butterfly)	Bent-arm fly
3	Back	12-15	3	Bent over row	Seated row	Rowing exercise
4	Shoulder	12-15	3	Standing press	Seated press	Shoulder press
5	Back	12-15	3	Dumbbell row	Lat pull-down	Pull-down/ pull-over exercise
6	Back of arm	12-15	3	Dumbbell triceps extension	Triceps push-down	Triceps extension
7	Front of arm	12-15	3	Biceps curl	Low pulley curl	Preacher curl
8	Thigh	12-15	3	Lunge	Leg press	Dual leg press
9	Abdomen	15-25	3	Trunk curl	Trunk curl	Trunk curl
10	Calf	12-15	3	Standing calf raise	Heel raise	Heel raise

REST PERIOD: 30 seconds
COOL-DOWN: Slow walking for 5 minutes, then stretching
APPROXIMATE CALORIES EXPENDED: 405-435

WORKOUT TIPS

Because this program contains two chest exercises listed in order, you may need to readjust the load you are using in exercise 2 to successfully complete three back-to-back sets.

BODY SHAPING

TOTAL TIME: 1 hour, 4 minutes

WEEKS: 1 and 2
DAYS OF THE WEEK: 2 nonconsecutive days
WARM-UP: Easy jogging or rope skipping for 5 minutes, then stretching

UPPER BODY EXERCISES: 34 minutes

#	Muscle group	Reps	Sets	Free weight	Pivot machine	Cam machine
1	Chest	10-12	3	Bench press	Bench press	Chest press
2	Chest	10-12	2	Dumbbell fly	Pec deck (butterfly)	Bent-arm fly
3	Back	10-12	2	Bent over row	Seated row	Rowing exercise
4	Shoulder	10-12	3	Standing press	Seated press	Shoulder press
5	Back	10-12	2	Dumbbell row	Lat pull-down	Pull-down/pull-over exercise
6	Back of arm	10-12	2	Dumbbell triceps extension	Triceps push-down	Triceps extension
7	Front of arm	10-12	2	Biceps curl	Low pulley curl	Preacher curl

REST PERIOD: 1 minute
COOL-DOWN: Slow walking for 5 minutes, then stretching
APPROXIMATE CALORIES EXPENDED: 350-380

WORKOUT TIPS

Be sure to perform the new exercises (2 and 5) back-to-back and in the order listed above.

BODY SHAPING

TOTAL TIME: 1 hour, 7 minutes

WEEKS: 1 and 2
DAYS OF THE WEEK: 2 nonconsecutive days
WARM-UP: Easy jogging or rope skipping for 5 minutes,
then stretching

LOWER BODY EXERCISES: 37 minutes

#	Muscle group	Reps	Sets	Free weight	Pivot machine	Cam machine
1	Thigh	10-12	3	Squat	Leg press	Dual leg press
2	Thigh	10-12	3	Lunge	Horizontal leg press	Horizontal leg press
3	Back of thigh	10-12	2	Leg curl	Leg curl	Leg curl
4	Front of thigh	10-12	2	Leg extension	Leg extension	Leg extension
5	Calf	10-12	2	Standing calf raise	Heel raise	Heel raise
6	Abdomen	15-25	3	Trunk curl	Trunk curl	Trunk curl

REST PERIOD: 1 minute
COOL-DOWN: Slow walking for 5 minutes, then stretching
APPROXIMATE CALORIES EXPENDED: 335-365

WORKOUT TIPS

Be sure to perform the new exercises (1, 3, 4, and 5) back-to-back
and in the order listed above.

BODY SHAPING

TOTAL TIME: 1 hour, 12 minutes

WEEKS: 3 and 4
DAYS OF THE WEEK: 2 nonconsecutive days
WARM-UP: Easy jogging or rope skipping for 5 minutes, then stretching

UPPER BODY EXERCISES: 42 minutes

#	Muscle group	Reps	Sets	Free weight	Pivot machine	Cam machine
1	Chest	10-12	3	Bench press	Bench press	Chest press
2	Chest	10-12	3	Dumbbell fly	Pec deck (butterfly)	Bent-arm fly
3	Back	10-12	3	Bent over row	Seated row	Rowing exercise
4	Shoulder	10-12	3	Standing press	Seated press	Shoulder press
5	Back	10-12	3	Dumbbell row	Lat pull-down	Pull-down/pull-over exercise
6	Back of arm	10-12	3	Dumbbell triceps extension	Triceps push-down	Triceps extension
7	Front of arm	10-12	3	Biceps curl	Low pulley curl	Preacher curl

REST PERIOD: 1 minute
COOL-DOWN: Slow walking for 5 minutes, then stretching
APPROXIMATE CALORIES EXPENDED: 420-450

WORKOUT TIPS

Because this program contains two chest exercises listed in order, you may need to readjust the load you are using in exercise 2 to successfully complete three back-to-back sets.

BODY SHAPING

TOTAL TIME: 1 hour, 7 minutes

WEEKS: 3 and 4
DAYS OF THE WEEK: 2 nonconsecutive days
WARM-UP: Easy jogging or rope skipping for 5 minutes,
   then stretching

LOWER BODY EXERCISES: 39 minutes

#	Muscle group	Reps	Sets	Free weight	Pivot machine	Cam machine
1	Thigh	10-12	3	Squat	Leg press	Dual leg press
2	Thigh	10-12	3	Lunge	Horizontal leg press	Horizontal leg press
3	Back of thigh	10-12	3	Leg curl	Leg curl	Leg curl
4	Front of thigh	10-12	3	Leg extension	Leg extension	Leg extension
5	Calf	10-12	3	Standing calf raise	Heel raise	Heel raise
6	Abdomen	15-25	3	Trunk curl	Trunk curl	Trunk curl

REST PERIOD: 1 minute
COOL-DOWN: Slow walking for 5 minutes, then stretching
APPROXIMATE CALORIES EXPENDED: 375-405

WORKOUT TIPS

Because this program contains two thigh exercises listed in order,
you may need to readjust the load you are using in exercise 2 to
successfully complete three back-to-back sets.

TOTAL TIME: 1 hour, 18 minutes

WEEKS: 1 and 2

DAYS OF THE WEEK: 2 nonconsecutive days

WARM-UP: Easy jogging or rope skipping for 5 minutes, then stretching. Before performing your first set of exercises 1 and 4, do one warm-up set of 8 to 10 repetitions with half to three quarters of the load you typically use for that exercise. Rest 1 to 2 minutes before starting your scheduled sets.

UPPER BODY EXERCISES: 48 minutes

#	Muscle group	Reps	Sets	Free weight	Machine pivot	Machine cam
1	Chest	6-8	3	Bench press	Bench press	Chest press
2	Chest	8-10	3	Dumbbell fly	Pec deck (butterfly)	Bent-arm fly
3	Back	8-10	3	Bent over row	Seated row	Rowing exercise
4	Shoulder	6-8	3	Standing press	Seated press	Shoulder press
5	Back	8-10	3	Dumbbell row	Lat pull-down	Pull-down/ pull-over exercise
6	Back of arm	8-10	3	Dumbbell triceps extension	Triceps push-down	Triceps extension
7	Front of arm	8-10	3	Biceps curl	Low pulley curl	Preacher curl

REST PERIOD: 2 minutes for exercises 1 and 4; 1 minute for all others

COOL-DOWN: Slow walking for 5 minutes, then stretching

APPROXIMATE CALORIES EXPENDED: 475-505

WORKOUT TIPS

In exercises 1 and 4 you will perform 6 to 8 reps. To do this add 5 to 10 pounds to the loads from the Yellow zone or consult chapter 12 for a more specific method for determining new loads. Notice that the heavier sets of 6 to 8 repetitions require more rest between sets.

STRENGTH TRAINING

**W
O
R
K
O
U
T**

TOTAL TIME: 1 hour, 9 minutes

WEEKS: 1 and 2

DAYS OF THE WEEK: 2 nonconsecutive days

WARM-UP: Easy jogging or rope skipping for 5 minutes, then stretching. Before performing your first set of exercise 1, do one warm-up set of 8 to 10 repetitions with half to three quarters of the load you typically use for that exercise. Rest 1 to 2 minutes before starting your scheduled sets.

LOWER BODY EXERCISES: 44 minutes

#	Muscle group	Reps	Sets	Free weight	Pivot machine	Cam machine
1	Thigh	6-8	3	Squat	Leg press	Dual leg press
2	Thigh	8-10	3	Lunge	Horizontal leg press	Horizontal leg press
3	Back of thigh	8-10	3	Leg curl	Leg curl	Leg curl
4	Front of thigh	8-10	3	Leg extension	Leg extension	Leg extension
5	Calf	8-10	3	Standing calf raise	Heel raise	Heel raise
6	Abdomen	15-25	3	Trunk curl	Trunk curl	Trunk curl

REST PERIOD: 2 minutes for exercise 1, 1 minute for all others

COOL-DOWN: Slow walking for 5 minutes, then stretching

APPROXIMATE CALORIES EXPENDED: 390-420

WORKOUT TIPS

In exercise 1 you will perform 6 to 8 reps. To do this add 10 to 20 pounds to the loads from the Yellow zone or consult chapter 12 for a more specific method for determining new loads. Notice that the heavier sets of 6 to 8 repetitions require more rest between sets.

STRENGTH TRAINING

TOTAL TIME: 1 hour, 23 minutes

WEEKS: 3 and 4

DAYS OF THE WEEK: 2 nonconsecutive days

WARM-UP: Easy jogging or rope skipping for 5 minutes, then stretching. Before performing your first set of exercises 1 and 4, do one warm-up set of 8 to 10 repetitions with half to three quarters of the load you typically use for that exercise. Rest 1 to 2 minutes before starting your scheduled sets.

UPPER BODY EXERCISES: 53 minutes

#	Muscle group	Reps	Sets	Free weight	Pivot machine	Cam machine
1	Chest	6-8	4	Bench press	Bench press	Chest press
2	Chest	8-10	3	Dumbbell fly	Pec deck (butterfly)	Bent-arm fly
3	Back	8-10	3	Bent over row	Seated row	Rowing exercise
4	Shoulder	6-8	4	Standing press	Seated press	Shoulder press
5	Back	8-10	3	Dumbbell row	Lat pull-down	Pull-down/pull-over exercise
6	Back of arm	8-10	3	Dumbbell triceps extension	Triceps push-down	Triceps extension
7	Front of arm	8-10	3	Biceps curl	Low pulley curl	Preacher curl

REST PERIOD: 2 minutes for exercises 1 and 4; 1 minute for all others

COOL-DOWN: Slow walking for 5 minutes, then stretching

APPROXIMATE CALORIES EXPENDED: 520-550

WORKOUT TIPS

As you begin performing four sets in exercises 1 and 4, you may have to decrease the load by 5 pounds to successfully complete all four sets.

STRENGTH TRAINING

4 WORKOUT

TOTAL TIME: 1 hour, 14 minutes

WEEKS: 3 and 4

DAYS OF THE WEEK: 2 nonconsecutive days

WARM-UP: Easy jogging or rope skipping for 5 minutes, then stretching. Before performing your first set of exercise 1, do one warm-up set of 8 to 10 repetitions with half to three quarters of the load you typically use for that exercise. Rest 1 to 2 minutes before starting your scheduled sets.

LOWER BODY EXERCISES: 33 minutes

#	Muscle group	Reps	Sets	Free weight	Pivot machine	Cam machine
1	Thigh	6-8	4	Squat	Leg press	Dual leg press
2	Thigh	8-10	3	Lunge	Horizontal leg press	Horizontal leg press
3	Back of thigh	8-10	3	Leg curl	Leg curl	Leg curl
4	Front of thigh	8-10	3	Leg extension	Leg extension	Leg extension
5	Calf	8-10	3	Standing calf raise	Heel raise	Heel raise
6	Abdomen	15-25	3	Trunk curl	Trunk curl	Trunk curl

REST PERIOD: 2 minutes for exercise 1; 1 minute for all others

COOL-DOWN: Slow walking for 5 minutes, then stretching

APPROXIMATE CALORIES EXPENDED: 435-465

WORKOUT TIPS

As you begin performing four sets in exercise 1, you may have to decrease the load by 10 pounds to successfully complete all four sets.

11

Red Zone

The Red zone is for you if you have been weight training recently on a consistent basis and scored in the "High" fitness classification from chapter 3 or if you completed the Orange zone and are looking for a more advanced program. The workouts in this zone represent a serious commitment to following an advanced program.

Zone Highlights

The Red zone uses four 1-week training periods for each training outcome. If there are any exercises you have never performed or if you are unsure about the correct exercise techniques, please refer to Appendix A or consult a professional. Remember to use a spotter for free weight exercises that require one.

- The **muscle toning** program includes three to four sets of 12 to 15 reps in 10 exercises for three workouts a week. There's one exercise for each major muscle group (except where noted): chest (two exercises), back (two exercises), shoulders, biceps, triceps, thighs, calves, and abdomen.
- The **body shaping** program continues to add sets to the 4 training days (2 upper body and 2 lower body) per week; you will perform three to four sets of 10 to 12 reps in each of your seven upper body and six lower body exercises. The upper body exercises include two each for the chest and back and one for the shoulders, the biceps,

and the triceps. The lower body exercises include two for the thighs and one for the back of the thigh (hamstrings), the front of the thigh (quadriceps), the calves, and the abdomen.

- The **strength training** program includes two upper body and two lower body workouts each week using the same exercises as the body shaping program. However, depending upon the exercise, the program now has different repetition goals: 4 to 6 reps (for weeks 1 and 2) and 2 to 4 reps (for weeks 3 and 4) for the major or core exercises and 8 to 10 for all others. In this zone you will begin performing weight-lifting exercises as part of your warm-up. Follow the warm-up procedure outlined in the warm-up section of each strength training workout. Warm-up sets are not counted in the number of sets you are scheduled to complete. During this zone, you will complete four sets in the core exercises and three sets in all the others.

Choosing Your Training Days

It is important not to weight train the same muscle group on 2 consecutive days or, on the other hand, to allow more than 3 days to go by between sessions. In either case you would be compromising your improvements. So, for the muscle toning workouts you might follow a Monday/ Wednesday/Friday or a Tuesday/Thursday/Saturday schedule.

To determine the most effective way to complete four body shaping or strength training sessions per week, simply choose from the following table one of the three options for your training days. Choose an option that you can stick to consistently and that is convenient for you. Each option provides two workouts each for your upper and lower body and distributes all of the workouts so that you have sufficient rest days between similar weight training sessions.

Training day option	Upper body workouts	Lower body workouts
1	Mondays and Thursdays	Tuesdays and Fridays
2	Sundays and Wednesdays	Mondays and Thursdays
3	Tuesdays and Fridays	Wednesdays and Saturdays

MUSCLE TONING

TOTAL TIME: 1 hour, 17 minutes

WEEKS: 1 and 2
DAYS OF THE WEEK: 3 nonconsecutive days
WARM-UP: Easy jogging or rope skipping for 5 minutes, then stretching

EXERCISES: 47 minutes

#	Muscle group	Reps	Sets	Free weight	Pivot machine	Cam machine
1	Chest	12-15	4	Bench press	Bench press	Chest press
2	Chest	12-15	3	Dumbbell fly	Pec deck (butterfly)	Bent-arm fly
3	Back	12-15	4	Bent over row	Seated row	Rowing exercise
4	Shoulder	12-15	4	Standing press	Seated press	Shoulder press
5	Back	12-15	3	Dumbbell row	Lat pull-down	Pull-down/pull-over exercise
6	Back of arm	12-15	4	Dumbbell triceps extension	Triceps push-down	Triceps extension
7	Front of arm	12-15	4	Biceps curl	Low pulley curl	Preacher curl
8	Thigh	12-15	4	Lunge	Leg press	Dual leg press
9	Abdomen	15-25	4	Trunk curl	Trunk curl	Trunk curl
10	Calf	12-15	3	Standing calf raise	Heel raise	Heel raise

REST PERIOD: 30 seconds
COOL-DOWN: Slow walking for 5 minutes, then stretching
APPROXIMATE CALORIES EXPENDED: 470-500

WORKOUT TIPS

As you begin performing four sets in your major exercises, you may have to slightly decrease the load (5 pounds upper body, 10 pounds lower body) to allow you to successfully complete all four sets.

MUSCLE TONING

2 **WORKOUT**

TOTAL TIME: 1 hour, 20 minutes

WEEKS: 3 and 4
DAYS OF THE WEEK: 3 nonconsecutive days
WARM-UP: Easy jogging or rope skipping for 5
minutes, then stretching

EXERCISES: 50 minutes

#	Muscle group	Reps	Sets	Free weight	Pivot machine	Cam machine
1	Chest	12-15	4	Bench press	Bench press	Chest press
2	Chest	12-15	4	Dumbbell fly	Pec deck (butterfly)	Bent-arm fly
3	Back	12-15	4	Bent over row	Seated row	Rowing exercise
4	Shoulder	12-15	4	Standing press	Seated press	Shoulder press
5	Back	12-15	4	Dumbbell row	Lat pull-down	Pull-down/ pull-over exercise
6	Back of arm	12-15	4	Dumbbell triceps extension	Triceps push-down	Triceps extension
7	Front of arm	12-15	4	Biceps curl	Low pulley curl	Preacher curl
8	Thigh	12-15	4	Lunge	Leg press	Dual leg press
9	Abdomen	15-25	4	Trunk curl	Trunk curl	Trunk curl
10	Calf	12-15	4	Standing calf raise	Heel raise	Heel raise

REST PERIOD: 30 seconds
COOL-DOWN: Slow walking for 5 minutes, then stretching
APPROXIMATE CALORIES EXPENDED: 495-525

WORKOUT TIPS

When increasing your workout loads, you do not have to add
weight to all four sets; treat each set individually when you apply
the 2-for-2 rule.

BODY SHAPING

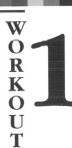
TOTAL TIME: 1 hour, 15 minutes

WEEKS: 1 and 2

DAYS OF THE WEEK: 2 nonconsecutive days

WARM-UP: Easy jogging or rope skipping for 5 minutes, then stretching

UPPER BODY EXERCISES: 45 minutes

#	Muscle group	Reps	Sets	Free weight	Pivot machine	Cam machine
1	Chest	10-12	4	Bench press	Bench press	Chest press
2	Chest	10-12	3	Dumbbell fly	Pec deck (butterfly)	Bent-arm fly
3	Back	10-12	3	Bent over row	Seated row	Rowing exercise
4	Shoulder	10-12	4	Standing press	Seated press	Shoulder press
5	Back	10-12	3	Dumbbell row	Lat pull-down	Pull-down/pull-over exercise
6	Back of arm	10-12	3	Dumbbell triceps extension	Triceps push-down	Triceps extension
7	Front of arm	10-12	3	Biceps curl	Low pulley curl	Preacher curl

REST PERIOD: 1 minute

COOL-DOWN: Slow walking for 5 minutes, then stretching

APPROXIMATE CALORIES EXPENDED: 445-475

WORKOUT TIPS

As you begin performing four sets in exercises 1 and 4, you may have to slightly decrease the load (5 pounds) in order to successfully complete all four sets.

BODY SHAPING

2 W O R K O U T

TOTAL TIME: 1 hour, 12 minutes

WEEKS: 1 and 2
DAYS OF THE WEEK: 2 nonconsecutive days
WARM-UP: Easy jogging or rope skipping for 5 minutes, then stretching

LOWER BODY EXERCISES: 42 minutes

#	Muscle group	Reps	Sets	Free weight	Pivot machine	Cam machine
1	Thigh	10-12	4	Squat	Leg press	Dual leg press
2	Thigh	10-12	4	Lunge	Horizontal leg press	Horizontal leg press
3	Back of thigh	10-12	3	Leg curl	Leg curl	Leg curl
4	Front of thigh	10-12	3	Leg extension	Leg extension	Leg extension
5	Calf	10-12	3	Standing calf raise	Heel raise	Heel raise
6	Abdomen	15-25	4	Trunk curl	Trunk curl	Trunk curl

REST PERIOD: 1 minute
COOL-DOWN: Slow walking for 5 minutes, then stretching
APPROXIMATE CALORIES EXPENDED: 420-450

WORKOUT TIPS

As you begin performing four sets in exercises 1 and 2, you may have to slightly decrease the load (10 pounds) in order to successfully complete all four sets.

BODY SHAPING

TOTAL TIME: 1 hour, 22 minutes

WEEKS: 3 and 4
DAYS OF THE WEEK: 2 nonconsecutive days
WARM-UP: Easy jogging or rope skipping for 5 minutes, then stretching

UPPER BODY EXERCISES: 52 minutes

#	Muscle group	Reps	Sets	Free weight	Pivot machine	Cam machine
1	Chest	10-12	4	Bench press	Bench press	Chest press
2	Chest	10-12	4	Dumbbell fly	Pec deck (butterfly)	Bent-arm fly
3	Back	10-12	4	Bent over row	Seated row	Rowing exercise
4	Shoulder	10-12	4	Standing press	Seated press	Shoulder press
5	Back	10-12	4	Dumbbell row	Lat pull-down	Pull-down/ pull-over exercise
6	Back of arm	10-12	4	Dumbbell triceps extension	Triceps push-down	Triceps extension
7	Front of arm	10-12	4	Biceps curl	Low pulley curl	Preacher curl

REST PERIOD: 1 minute
COOL-DOWN: Slow walking for 5 minutes, then stretching
APPROXIMATE CALORIES EXPENDED: 515-545

WORKOUT TIPS

When increasing your workout loads, you do not have to add weight to all four sets; treat each set individually when you apply the 2-for-2 rule.

BODY SHAPING

W O R K O U T

TOTAL TIME: 1 hour, 16 minutes

WEEKS: 3 and 4
DAYS OF THE WEEK: 2 nonconsecutive days
WARM-UP: Easy jogging or rope skipping for 5 minutes, then stretching

LOWER BODY EXERCISES: 46 minutes

#	Muscle group	Reps	Sets	Free weight	Pivot machine	Cam machine
1	Thigh	10-12	4	Squat	Leg press	Dual leg press
2	Thigh	10-12	4	Lunge	Horizontal leg press	Horizontal leg press
3	Back of thigh	10-12	4	Leg curl	Leg curl	Leg curl
4	Front of thigh	10-12	4	Leg extension	Leg extension	Leg extension
5	Calf	10-12	4	Standing calf raise	Heel raise	Heel raise
6	Abdomen	15-25	4	Trunk curl	Trunk curl	Trunk curl

REST PERIOD: 1 minute
COOL-DOWN: Slow walking for 5 minutes, then stretching
APPROXIMATE CALORIES EXPENDED: 460-490

WORKOUT TIPS

When increasing your workout loads, you do not have to add weight to all four sets; treat each set individually when you apply the 2-for-2 rule.

STRENGTH TRAINING

TOTAL TIME: 1 hour, 31 minutes

WEEKS: 1 and 2

DAYS OF THE WEEK: 2 nonconsecutive days

WARM-UP: Easy jogging or rope skipping for 5 minutes, then stretching. Before performing your first set of exercises 1 and 4, do two warm-up sets of 8 to 10 and 4 to 6 repetitions with half and three quarters, respectively, of the load you typically use for that exercise. Rest 1 to 3 minutes before starting your scheduled sets.

UPPER BODY EXERCISES: 34 minutes

#	Muscle group	Reps	Sets	Free weight	Pivot machine	Cam machine
1	Chest	4-6	4	Bench press	Bench press	Chest press
2	Chest	8-10	3	Dumbbell fly	Pec deck (butterfly)	Bent-arm fly
3	Back	8-10	3	Bent over row	Seated row	Rowing exercise
4	Shoulder	4-6	4	Standing press	Seated press	Shoulder press
5	Back	8 10	3	Dumbbell row	Lat pull-down	Pull-down/ pull-over exercise
6	Back of arm	8-10	3	Dumbbell triceps extension	Triceps push-down	Triceps extension
7	Front of arm	8-10	3	Biceps curl	Low pulley curl	Preacher curl

REST PERIOD: 3 minutes for exercises 1 and 4; 1 minute for all others.

COOL-DOWN: Slow walking for 5 minutes, then stretching

APPROXIMATE CALORIES EXPENDED: 590-620

WORKOUT TIPS

In exercises 1 and 4 you will perform 4 to 6 reps. To do this add 5 to 10 pounds to the loads from the Orange zone or consult chapter 12 for a more specific method for determining new loads. Notice that the heavier sets of 4 to 6 repetitions require more rest between sets.

2 WORKOUT

TOTAL TIME: 1 hour, 22 minutes

WEEKS: 1 and 2

DAYS OF THE WEEK: 2 nonconsecutive days

WARM-UP: Easy jogging or rope skipping for 5 minutes, then stretching. Before performing your first set of exercise 1, do two warm-up sets of 8 to 10 and 4 to 6 repetitions with half and three quarters, respectively, of the load you typically use for that exercise. Rest 1 to 3 minutes before starting your scheduled sets.

LOWER BODY EXERCISES: 52 minutes

#	Muscle group	Reps	Sets	Free weight	Pivot machine	Cam machine
1	Thigh	4-6	4	Squat	Leg press	Dual leg press
2	Thigh	8-10	3	Lunge	Horizontal leg press	Horizontal leg press
3	Back of thigh	8-10	3	Leg curl	Leg curl	Leg curl
4	Front of thigh	8-10	3	Leg extension	Leg extension	Leg extension
5	Calf	8-10	3	Standing calf raise	Heel raise	Heel raise
6	Abdomen	15-25	3	Trunk curl	Trunk curl	Trunk curl

REST PERIOD: 3 minutes for exercise 1, 1 minute for all others.

COOL-DOWN: Slow walking for 5 minutes, then stretching

APPROXIMATE CALORIES EXPENDED: 510-540

WORKOUT TIPS

In exercise 1 you will perform 4 to 6 reps. To do this add 10 to 20 pounds to the loads from the Orange zone or consult chapter 12 for a more specific method for determining new loads. Notice that the heavier sets of 4 to 6 repetitions require more rest between sets.

STRENGTH TRAINING

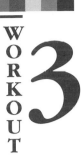
TOTAL TIME: 1 hour, 39 minutes

WEEKS: 3 and 4

DAYS OF THE WEEK: 2 nonconsecutive days

WARM-UP: Easy jogging or rope skipping for 5 minutes, then stretching. Before performing your first set of exercises 1 and 4, do three warm-up sets of 8 to 10, 6 to 8, and 4 to 6 repetitions with one half, two thirds, and three quarters, respectively, of the load you typically use for that exercise. Rest 1 to 4 minutes before starting your scheduled sets.

UPPER BODY EXERCISES: 1 hour, 9 minutes

#	Muscle group	Reps	Sets	Free weight	Pivot machine	Cam machine
1	Chest	2-4	4	Bench press	Bench press	Chest press
2	Chest	8-10	3	Dumbbell fly	Pec deck (butterfly)	Bent-arm fly
3	Back	8-10	3	Bent over row	Seated row	Rowing exercise
4	Shoulder	2-4	4	Standing press	Seated press	Shoulder press
5	Back	8-10	3	Dumbbell row	Lat pull-down	Pull-down/ pull-over exercise
6	Back of arm	8-10	3	Dumbbell triceps extension	Triceps push-down	Triceps extension
7	Front of arm	8-10	3	Biceps curl	Low pulley curl	Preacher curl

REST PERIOD: 4 minutes for exercises 1 and 4; 1 minute for all others.

COOL-DOWN: Slow walking for 5 minutes, then stretching

APPROXIMATE CALORIES EXPENDED: 665-695

WORKOUT TIPS

In exercises 1 and 4 you will perform 2 to 4 reps. To do this add 5 to 10 pounds to the loads from week 1 or consult chapter 12 for a more specific method for determining new loads. Notice that the heavier sets of 2 to 4 repetitions require more rest between sets.

4 WORKOUT

TOTAL TIME: 1 hour, 30 minutes

WEEKS: 3 and 4
DAYS OF THE WEEK: 2 nonconsecutive days
WARM-UP: Easy jogging or rope skipping for 5 minutes, then stretching. Before performing your first set of exercise 1, do three warm-up sets of 8 to 10, 6 to 8, and 4 to 6 repetitions with one half, two thirds, and three quarters, respectively, of the load you typically use for that exercise. Rest 1 to 4 minutes before starting your scheduled sets.

LOWER BODY EXERCISES: 1 hour

#	Muscle group	Reps	Sets	Free weight	Pivot machine	Cam machine
1	Thigh	2-4	4	Squat	Leg press	Dual leg press
2	Thigh	8-10	3	Lunge	Horizontal leg press	Horizontal leg press
3	Back of thigh	8-10	3	Leg curl	Leg curl	Leg curl
4	Front of thigh	8-10	3	Leg extension	Leg extension	Leg extension
5	Calf	8-10	3	Standing calf raise	Heel raise	Heel raise
6	Abdomen	15-25	3	Trunk curl	Trunk curl	Trunk curl

REST PERIOD: 4 minutes for exercise 1; 1 minute for all others.
COOL-DOWN: Slow walking for 5 minutes, then stretching
APPROXIMATE CALORIES EXPENDED: 585-615

WORKOUT TIPS

In exercise 1 you will perform 2 to 4 reps. To do this add 10 to 20 pounds to the load from week 2 or consult chapter 12 for a more specific method for determining new loads. Notice that the heavier sets of 2 to 4 repetitions require more rest between sets.

PART III

TRAINING BY THE WORKOUT ZONES

Now that you've been introduced to the workouts themselves, the chapters in this part will provide guidance on how to use them. When you've finished reading these chapters, you will have the knowledge and confidence to follow the program we suggest or any that you design.

If you choose to follow the program we've created, then most of the planning has been done for you. Use the following pages to determine your training loads and to learn how to make load adjustments. If you want to design your own program, you'll find guidelines for that here too.

Chapter 13 outlines the program you can follow, showing the progression through the zones and the days on which you should weight train. We've offered guidelines for cross-training too and have provided sample programs for you to follow.

The final chapter explains how to chart your training progress, and it provides some guidance on how to establish your short- and long-term goals and how to recognize when you've met those goals.

12

Setting Up Your Program

This chapter "walks" you through procedures to follow as you prepare to weight train. Should you decide to develop your own workouts, we've also included guidelines for you to use—the same guidelines that were used to develop the workouts in chapters 6 through 11. These guidelines will make designing your own program relatively easy.

Filling in Your Workout Chart

If you have ever observed people who are in great training shape, you will invariably see them recording information on a chart or a booklet. This is a very important part of being successful in your training, because it helps you maintain your interest, allows you to see improvement, and helps you to establish reasonable goals. To fill in your workout chart, follow the four steps presented here.

Step 1. Locate the Workouts

After determining which zone you plan to work in, locate the workouts in that zone for your desired training outcome. Note that some are 2-day-a-week programs and others are 3- and 4-day-a-week programs.

Step 2. Make Copies of Workout Chart

At the top of the page of the workouts you selected in Step 1 you'll see the number of days (per week) you'll weight train. Find the correct workout chart in Appendix B according to whether you'll train 2, 3, or 4 days each week.

For the body shaping and strength training outcomes, notice that when the upper body and lower body workouts are separated into two different days in the later zones, you will complete each workout twice a week for a total of 4 training days.

Photocopy the workout chart that matches the number of days listed for the workout zone. Each chart covers a 1-week period of training while each workout zone covers a 4-week period; so you will need to make at least four copies of the chart. If you plan to follow the workout longer than 4 weeks, make an appropriate number of copies of this chart. As you progress from one zone to another, follow the same procedure.

Step 3. Select and Record Exercises

After considering the equipment available to you and your familiarity with its use, decide which type you will use and record the exercise names onto the workout chart. Notice that each workout zone includes exercises for free weight and two types of machines (from which to select single- and multi-unit pivot and cam machines). If you are inexperienced you should begin with machine exercises. Free weight exercises require more skill than machine exercises and sometimes require a spotter(s). In each workout, notice that to the left of each exercise is the muscle group that is "worked" by that exercise. Knowing the muscle group enables you to select an alternative exercise to replace one that you may not be able to perform because the equipment needed is not available. Record the exercises you will perform in the "Exercises" column of the workout chart. Remember, if you are not familiar with the exercises listed, refer to Appendix A.

Step 4. Record Sets and Repetitions

Refer to the set and repetition information included in the selected workout, and transfer these numbers onto the workout chart in the "Sets/ Reps" column. Be sure to record the set and repetition information into the correct week.

Your workout chart provides a "diary" of each training day. Be sure to record all the information requested so you'll be able to easily recognize the successes that occur as you train on a regular basis.

Filling in Your Cross-Training Workout Chart

If you plan to cross-train, use a cross-training workout chart in Appendix B to merge aerobic activity intervals with your weight training program. Remember, all of the exercises, their numbers of sets and repetitions, and the number of workouts per week remain as they are shown in the workout zones.

Follow the four steps outlined above, but also fill in your choice of aerobic exercises on the cross-training workout chart:

1. Determine (see chapter 13) your THR range and write it in the space at the bottom of the chart.
2. Write in the name of an appropriate type of aerobic exercise (see chapter 13) in the space marked "aerobic exercise."
3. Take your heart rate after completing the last aerobic interval and write it on the workout sheet.

Determining Training Loads

Determining a load or weight that you can lift for the required number of repetitions listed in the chapter workouts is a real challenge. What follows is a description of two methods to help you accomplish this task. If you are new to weight training and have no experience in selecting training loads, use the Green zone load guidelines. If you are experienced, use the Blue-Red zone load guidelines.

Green Zone Load Guidelines

Table 12.1 is a load-calculation table that will help you establish appropriate training loads for workouts in the Green zone. Use these steps when establishing loads:

1. Look at the exercise names you recorded on your workout chart, and then circle the corresponding coefficients on the table. Notice that men and women use different coefficient values.
2. Record your body weight in the blank in the far left-hand column (labeled BWT) next to the coefficient column. *Important:* Men weighing 175 pounds or more and women weighing 140 pounds or more should record 175 and 140, respectively, for their body weight in the BWT column.
3. To determine what is referred to as the "trial load," multiply your body weight by the coefficient value. The load is called a "trial load" because you are trying it out to see if it will result in the required number of repetitions.
4. Round off the trial load to the nearest 5-pound increment, or if using machines, select the closest weight stack plate.

Table 12.1
Load Calculation Table

		Women				Exercise			Men			
BWT	Coeff.	Trial load	Reps compl.	Adj.	Training load		BWT	Coeff.	Trial load	Reps compl.	Adj.	Training load
						CHEST						
___	× .35 = ___	___	___	___	___	Bench press (FW)	___	× .60 = ___	___	___	___	___
___	× .27 = ___	___	___	___	___	Bent-arm fly (CM)	___	× .55 = ___	___	___	___	___
___	× .27 = ___	___	___	___	___	Chest press (PM)	___	× .55 = ___	___	___	___	___
						BACK						
___	× .35 = ___	___	___	___	___	Bent over row (FW)	___	× .45 = ___	___	___	___	___
___	× .20 = ___	___	___	___	___	Seated row (CM)	___	× .40 = ___	___	___	___	___
___	× .20 = ___	___	___	___	___	Pull-over exercise (CM)	___	× .40 = ___	___	___	___	___
___	× .25 = ___	___	___	___	___	Seated row (PM)	___	× .45 = ___	___	___	___	___
						SHOULDERS						
___	× .22 = ___	___	___	___	___	Standing press (FW)	___	× .38 = ___	___	___	___	___
___	× .15 = ___	___	___	___	___	Seated press (PM)	___	× .35 = ___	___	___	___	___
___	× .25 = ___	___	___	___	___	Shoulder press (CM)	___	× .40 = ___	___	___	___	___
						BICEPS						
___	× .23 = ___	___	___	___	___	Biceps curl (FW)	___	× .30 = ___	___	___	___	___
___	× .12 = ___	___	___	___	___	Preacher curl (CM)	___	× .20 = ___	___	___	___	___
___	× .15 = ___	___	___	___	___	Low pulley curl (PM)	___	× .25 = ___	___	___	___	___

Table 12.1 (continued)

BWT	**Coeff.**	**Trial load**	**Reps compl.**	**Adj.**	**Training load**	**Exercise**	**BWT**	**Coeff.**	**Trial load**	**Reps compl.**	**Adj.**	**Training load**
	Women							**Men**				
						TRICEPS						
___	× .12 =	___	___	___	___	Triceps extension (FW)	___	× .21 =	___	___	___	___
___	× .13 =	___	___	___	___	Triceps extension (CM)	___	× .35 =	___	___	___	___
___	× .19 =	___	___	___	___	Triceps push-down (PM)	___	× .32 =	___	___	___	___
						LEGS						
	5 pounds each hand					Lunge (FW)		10 pounds each hand				
___	× 1.0 =	___	___	___	___	Dual leg press (CM)	___	× 1.3 =	___	___	___	___
___	× 1.0 =	___	___	___	___	Leg press (PM)	___	× 1.3 =	___	___	___	___
						ABDOMINALS						
		No load				Trunk curl			No load			
___	× .20 =	___	___	___	___	Trunk curl (CM)	___	× .20 =	___	___	___	___

FW = Free weights; CM = Cam machines; PM = single- or multi-unit pivot machines.

Below is an example of how to use Table 12.1 to establish a trial load. In this example, the bench press exercise is being used, and the coefficient associated with it is .35 (for women). The woman weighs 120 pounds, and the trial load when rounded off (from 42) equals 40 pounds.

Table 12.1
Load Calculation Table

BWT	Coeff.	Trial load	Reps compl.	Adj.	Training load	Exercise
			Women			CHEST
120	× .35 =	*40*	___	___	___	Bench press (FW)
___	× .27 =	___	___	___	___	Bent-arm fly (CM)
___	× .27 =	___	___	___	___	Chest press (PM)
						BACK
___	× .35 =	___	___	___	___	Bent over row (FW)
___	× .20 =	___	___	___	___	Seated row (CM)

Calculating the trial load.

Try Out the Trial Load. After warming up, perform as many repetitions as you can with the trial load and record that number in the "Reps compl(eted)" column. The trial load may be too heavy or too light for a training load.

Make Load Adjustments. If you were able to perform more than 15 reps or were not able to perform 12 reps, refer to the Load Adjustment Table 12.2. This table will enable you to identify the correct training load.

Table 12.2
Load Adjustment Table

Reps completed	Adjustment (in pounds)
<7	– 15
8-9	– 10
10-11	– 5
12-15	0
16-17	+ 5
18-19	+ 10
>20	+ 15

Below is an example of how to use the Load Calculation and Load Adjustment Tables to create an appropriate training load. In this example, a man needs to calculate his training load for the bench press. For men, the coefficient associated with this exercise is .60. The man's trial load equaled 100 pounds (rounded off), and he performed 9 reps (instead of 12-15) with this load. According to the Load Adjustment Table, completing 9 reps requires an adjustment of −10 pounds. So, in this example the man subtracts 10 pounds from the trial load in Table 12.1, yielding a training load of 90 pounds; he then records his calculated training load onto the Load Calculation Table to the right of the bench press exercise. This procedure is used with all the exercises included in the workouts listed in the Green Workout zone.

Table 12.1
Load Calculation Table

Exercise	BWT	Coeff.	Trial load	Reps compl.	Adj.	Training load
CHEST				Men		
Bench press (FW)	165 ×	.60 =	100	9	-10	90
Bent arm fly (CM)	_____ ×	.55 =	_____	_____	_____	_____
Chest press (PM)	_____ ×	.55 =	_____	_____	_____	_____

Using the load adjustment table.

Blue-Red Zone Load Guidelines

If you choose one of the more advanced workout zones, you should use the **1 R**epetition **M**aximum (1RM) method for determining loads for some of the exercises in your workout. This method is significantly more demanding than using the load guidelines presented for beginners in the Green zone, because the 1RM procedure requires the use of heavier weights. It involves using a maximum weight in a single all-out effort. This 1RM approach is appropriate only for use with exercises that involve large muscle groups, such as the chest, shoulders, and legs (referred to as core exercises). Attempting a 1RM in an exercise that recruits smaller muscle groups—such as the forearm, arm, neck, thigh, or back—increases your chances for injury, because such muscles and joints may not be able to withstand the physical stress of lifting maximal loads. Table 12.3 lists exercises in this book that you can safely perform using the 1RM approach (as long as you use proper procedures).

Table 12.3
Exercises Suitable for a 1RM Effort

Muscle group	Core exercises	Exercise equipment
Chest	Bench press	*FW, PM
	Chest press	CM
Shoulders	Standing press	*FW
	Seated press	PM
	Shoulder press	CM
Thighs	Squats	*FW

FW = Free weights; PM = Pivot machine; CM = Cam machine
*All free weight exercises listed require an experienced spotter!

1RM Procedure for Core Exercises. Essentially, your task involves starting with a light warm-up load and progressively adding weight until, after five or six sets, you arrive at your 1RM. To be safe, you should approach the 1RM keeping in mind (1) the correct use of exercise technique, (2) the careful selection of loads, (3) the use of 2-minute rest periods between attempts, and (4) the use of a qualified person for spotting (if the exercise requires it).

If you have never attempted a 1RM, don't try it without first consulting a qualified strength and conditioning professional. Some free weight exercises require a skilled spotter, and all exercises require a reasonable level of previous physical training. Unless you are totally confident in your ability to perform the exercise correctly or have access to a qualified professional who can teach you the proper techniques, *do not attempt to perform a 1RM!* Table 12.4 summarizes the procedures for establishing a 1RM for core exercises. Carefully follow these directions to identify your 1RM.

Using the 1RM to Establish Training Loads for Core Exercises. Establishing your 1RM is the first of two steps for determining a training load for core exercises. The second step involves the use of Table 12.5 in conjunction with the workout you plan to follow. Simply locate the "Goal repetitions" column heading, which tells you the number of reps to be performed, and then in the "1RM value" column, locate the poundage found for the 1RM. Where these two columns intersect is the training load poundage. If needed, round off the weight to the nearest 5 pound or nearest weight stack plate when using machines.

For example, imagine a person is following one of the strength training workouts. The goal reps for an exercise such as the seated press are listed as 6, and his 1RM in this exercise is 170 (line 15). The 6 to 7 reps column

Table 12.4
**Load Guidelines for Establishing the 1RM in Core Exercises
in Blue-Red Workout Zones**

Set #	Estimate of appropriate load or amount to add	Perform only this number of reps
1	Warm-up—You could perform 20 reps with this load but . . . Rest 2 or more minutes	12
2	You could perform 10 reps with this load, but . . . Rest 2 or more minutes	6
3	You could perform 5-6 reps with this load, but . . . Rest 2 or more minutes	3
4	Add 10 pounds Rest 2 or more minutes	1
5	Add 10 pounds Rest 2 or more minutes	1
*6	Add 10 pounds	1

*Continue adding 10 pounds as needed until you can no longer lift the weight. When failure occurs, reduce the load by 5 pounds, rest 2 or more minutes, and try to perform 1 repetition. Record the heaviest weight succeeded with as your 1RM.

and the 170 1RM value intersect at the number 136. When rounded off to the nearest 5 pounds, this individual establishes a training load of 135 for the seated press. This value is then entered on the workout chart.

Establishing Training Loads for Noncore Exercises. For those exercises listed in your workout that are not core exercises, try to identify a load that will result in the reps listed in Table 12.6.

Making Load Adjustments. Once loads have been determined for the various exercises, you'll commonly find that they are too heavy or too light and do not result in the desired number of reps. If you find that this happens in one or more exercises, complete the following procedures to make proper load adjustments.

Load Adjustment Procedure for Blue-Red Workout Zones.

1. Determine, locate, and circle the goal reps in the left-hand column of Table 12.7.
2. Beneath the heading "Reps completed," locate and circle the actual appropriate range.
3. Where the "Goal reps" row and "Reps completed" column intersect is the load adjustment.
4. To establish a new training load, subtract (–) or add (+) the poundage listed to the original load.

Table 12.5
Training Load Determination Table
for Blue-Red Workout Zones

Line #	1RM value	Goal repetitions					
		12-15	10-12	8-9	6-7	4-5	2-3
1	30	18	21	23	24	26	27
2	40	24	28	30	32	34	36
3	50	30	35	38	40	43	45
4	60	36	42	45	48	51	54
5	70	42	49	52	56	60	63
6	80	48	56	60	64	68	72
7	90	54	63	68	72	77	81
8	100	60	70	75	80	85	90
9	110	66	77	83	88	94	99
10	120	72	84	90	96	102	108
11	130	78	91	98	104	111	117
12	140	84	98	105	112	119	125
13	150	90	105	113	120	128	135
14	160	96	112	120	128	136	144
15	170	102	119	128	136	145	153
16	180	108	126	135	144	153	162
17	190	114	133	143	152	162	171
18	200	120	140	150	160	170	180
19	210	126	147	158	168	179	189
20	220	132	154	165	176	187	198
21	230	138	161	173	184	196	207
22	240	144	168	180	192	204	216
23	250	150	175	188	200	213	225
24	260	156	182	195	208	221	234
25	270	162	189	203	216	230	243
26	280	168	196	210	224	248	252
27	290	174	203	218	232	247	261
28	300	180	210	225	240	255	270
29	310	186	217	233	248	264	279
30	320	192	224	240	256	272	288
31	330	198	231	248	264	281	297
32	340	204	238	255	272	289	306
33	350	210	245	263	280	298	316
34	360	216	252	278	288	306	324
35	370	222	259	280	296	315	333
36	380	228	266	285	304	323	342
37	390	234	273	293	312	332	351
38	400	240	280	300	320	340	360
	1RM value	Training loads					

Table 12.6
Load Guidelines for Noncore Exercises

Outcome desired	Load selected should result in
Muscle toning	12-15 reps
Body shaping	10-12 reps
Strength training	8-10 reps

For example, an individual wants to complete 10 reps ("Goal reps") with 110 pounds, but he or she is able to perform 15 reps. As shown, the goal reps of 10 intersect the number 15 at +10 pounds. When 10 is added to the 110-pound load, the adjusted load equals 120 pounds. Remember, it is not uncommon to have to make several adjustments before you can establish an accurate training load.

Even after you've established an appropriate training load, your strength will continue to increase and you will need to adjust your loads. Use the 2-for-2 rule to determine when to make load adjustments.

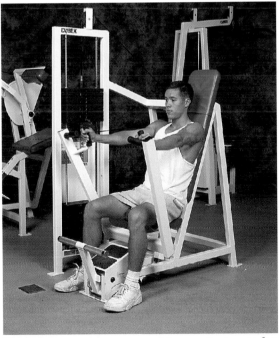

The chest press is an appropriate exercise to use for performing a 1RM on a machine.

The 2-for-2 Rule

As your strength increases as a natural outcome of training, use what is referred to as the 2-for-2 rule to make load adjustments. You should increase loads when you are able to perform 2 (or more) repetitions beyond the number listed in the last set for two consecutive workouts. For example, if you are supposed to perform 12 to 15 reps for two sets in an exercise and you complete 17 reps in the second set for 2 consecutive workout days, then you should increase the load. Add 10 pounds for your leg exercises and 5 on others, or refer to the Load Adjustment Table 12.2.

Designing Your Own Program

So, let's say you decide to design your own program. You may be in for a surprise, because designing a weight training program can be challenging; there are more variables that you probably realize. However, we have broken this process down into eight easy steps. If you want to gain a more in-depth understanding of how to design your own program, you should consult the books listed in the reference section of this book.

1. Establish Goals for Weight Training

The first step in designing your own program is to determine your goals for training. Some commonly sought goals for weight training include increases in muscular endurance, size, strength, and toning and improvements in the overall shape of your body. What are your goals? Decide on them now.

2. Select Exercises

After assessing your goals, you need to decide which exercises to include in your program. If your special interest is chest and arm development, then you need to include exercises that stress these muscle areas. You may decide to use the exercises included in chapters 6 through 11, or you may want to add additional exercises that for one reason or another you like. Regardless of the exercises you select, be sure to use loads that won't cause injury. Start light and add weight as needed to produce the reps you need. As you select each of your exercises, be sure to consider equipment, spotter requirements, and the amount of time you have to train.

3. Determine Training Frequency

After you have chosen your exercises, you need to decide how many days a week you will train. For beginners, 3 days a week is best. After you have trained a while you may wish to increase your workouts to four per week. Locate the appropriate workout chart in Appendix B based upon the number of days you intend to train and use it to record your workouts.

Table 12.7
Blue-Red Zone Load Adjustment Table

Goal reps	Reps completed with trial load									
	>18	16-17	14-15	12-13	10-11	8-9	6-7	4-5	2-3	<2
14-15	+10	+5		-5	-10	-15	-15	-20	-25	-30
12-13	+15	+10	+5		-5	-10	-15	-15	-20	-25
10-11	+15	+15	+10	+5		-5	-10	-15	-15	-20
8-9	+20	+15	+15	+10	+5		-5	-10	-15	-15
6-7	+25	+20	+15	+15	+10	+5		-5	-10	-15
4-5	+30	+25	+20	+15	+15	+10	+5		-5	-10
2-3	+35	+30	+25	+20	+20	+15	+10	+5		-5

Poundage increase (+) or decrease (−)

4. Arrange Exercises

Decisions on how you arrange exercises are very important, because they affect the intensity of training. You can use several different methods, such as exercising large muscle groups first (see Table 12.8) or alternating upper and lower body exercises (Table 12.9).

The most common arrangement is to alternate pushing with pulling exercises. With this method, you would follow a pushing exercise (like the bench press) with a pulling exercise (like the bent over row), or you might follow a pull exercise (like the biceps curl) with a push exercise (like the triceps press-down). Table 12.10 provides an example of this push-pull exercise arrangement. There is no one best method for everyone; sometimes the equipment available will determine your arrangement decisions. Whatever arrangement you select, try to avoid taxing the same muscle group again and again without allowing time for adequate recovery.

5. Determine Loads, Sets, and Repetitions

After arranging your exercises in an appropriate order, you need to determine what loads to use for each exercise. An exciting characteristic of weight training is that you can vary the loads, the number of sets, and

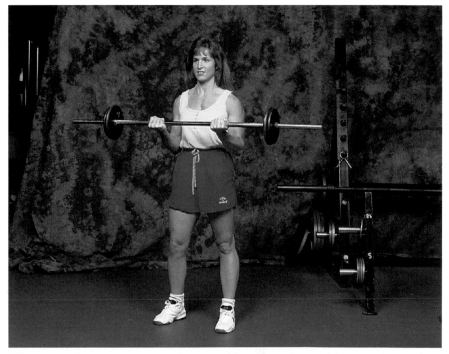

When arranging your own exercises, consider alternating pushing exercises with pulling exercises.

Table 12.8
Large to Small Muscle Group Arrangement

Exercise	Type (L/S)	Muscle group
Lunge	Large	Thigh and hip
Heel raise	Small	Calf
Bench press	Large	Chest
Triceps extension	Small	Arm (posterior)
Lat pull-down	Large	Upper back
Biceps curl	Small	Arm (anterior)

Table 12.9
Alternating Upper Body and Lower Body Exercises

Exercise	Type (UB/LB)	Muscle group
Bench press	Upper body	Chest
Lunge	Lower body	Thigh and hip
Biceps curl	Upper body	Arm (anterior)
Leg extension	Lower body	Thigh (anterior)
Standing press	Upper body	Shoulder
Leg curl	Lower body	Thigh (posterior)

Table 12.10
Alternating Push With Pull Exercises

Exercise	Type (PS/PL)	Muscle group
Bench press	Push	Chest
Lat pull-down	Pull	Back
Seated press	Push	Shoulder
Biceps curl	Pull	Arm (anterior)
Triceps extension	Push	Arm (posterior)
Leg curl	Pull	Thigh (posterior)
Leg extension	Push	Thigh (anterior)

the repetitions to produce the changes you want. Table 12.11 shows you how to achieve significant strength gains by using heavier loads with fewer repetitions (1-8) and performing three to five sets of the most important exercises. If you want muscle toning, you need to use lighter loads with many repetitions (12-20) and to include two to three sets of each exercise. This type of training program will also contribute to improvements in your cardiovascular fitness, if you integrate aerobic exercises with the weight training (as presented in chapter 13). If you want body shaping, you need to use moderate loads with a moderate number of

Table 12.11 Adjustments for Training Outcomes				
Relative loading	**Outcome of training**	**Rep range**	**# of sets**	**Rest between sets**
Light	Muscular toning	12-20	2-3	20-30 s
Moderate	Body shaping	8-12	3-6	30-90 s
Heavy	Strength training	1-8	3-5+	2-5 min

repetitions (8-12) and perform three to six sets. Combining a body shaping weight training program with sensible eating can bring about losses in body fat and increases in muscle—the end result being attractive changes to your body composition.

6. Determine Length of Rest Periods

Decide on the length of your rest periods between sets; this will vary depending on your training goals and your fitness level. Table 12.11 shows you how to plan longer rest periods for strength development, moderate rest periods for body shaping, and short rest periods for muscle toning.

7. Decide on Intensity of Training

As your training level improves, you may wish to increase the number of sets you perform in each exercise, the loads you use, and/or even the number of exercises. Decide on when and how you will make load increases. Typically, the more sets you perform of each exercise, the greater you'll improve. Thus, well-designed programs are built upon the proper selection of exercises, the amount of load, the number of sets and repetitions performed, the proper rest between exercises/sets, and the appropriate number of training days per week.

8. Consider Varying the Intensity of Your Program

As you become more skilled, you may want to modify your program by changing one or more of the variables just discussed. Experiment with different training approaches and find what works best for you. The most important factor is to train within your ability. Make your training decisions carefully; base them on your fitness level, experience, and training goals. Enjoy this time in your day, and feel good about your accomplishments and the contribution that weight training makes to your health and appearance.

13

Sample Weight Training Programs

This chapter presents sample programs that show you how to organize the workouts from Part II into a training schedule. For each training outcome, we'll show you how to organize your workouts on a weekly basis—days on which to train, days on which to rest, and how to progress through the zones. Next, we'll discuss the benefits of cross-training and show you how to add aerobic exercise to your weight training workouts.

Sample Weight Training Schedules

The sample programs on pages 127-129 show how to organize your training schedule for each weight training outcome: muscle toning, body shaping, and strength training. If muscle toning is your desired outcome, follow the schedule on page 127. If you plan to follow the body shaping program, use the schedule on page 128. If strength training is your desired outcome, follow the schedule on page 129.

Each line of the schedules represents a 2-week training period. For example, if your goal is muscle toning and you're working in the Green zone, you will perform Green workout 1 on Monday and Thursday of the first and second weeks, resting on the other days. In weeks 3 and 4, you'll perform Green workout 2 on Monday and Thursday. After working in the Green zone for 4 weeks, you have the option to move to the Blue zone or remain in the Green zone. If your score on the bench press test in chapter 3 indicated that you should start in a higher zone than the Green zone, simply begin following the sample program in the schedule that corresponds to the zone you're working in.

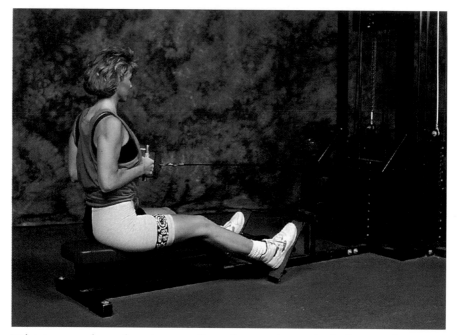

Make sure you know how to correctly perform each exercise before you begin.

Muscle Toning Program

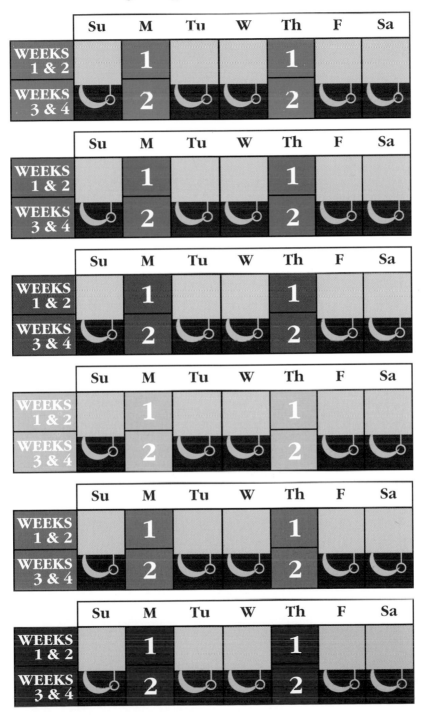

Body Shaping Program

	Su	M	Tu	W	Th	F	Sa
WEEKS 1 & 2		1		1		1	
WEEKS 3 & 4		2		2		2	

	Su	M	Tu	W	Th	F	Sa
WEEKS 1 & 2		1		1		1	
WEEKS 3 & 4		2		2		2	

	Su	M	Tu	W	Th	F	Sa
WEEKS 1 & 2		1		1		1	
WEEKS 3 & 4		2		2		2	

	Su	M	Tu	W	Th	F	Sa
WEEKS 1 & 2		1	2		1	2	
WEEKS 3 & 4		3	4		3	4	

	Su	M	Tu	W	Th	F	Sa
WEEKS 1 & 2		1	2		1	2	
WEEKS 3 & 4		3	4		3	4	

	Su	M	Tu	W	Th	F	Sa
WEEKS 1 & 2		1	2		1	2	
WEEKS 3 & 4		3	4		3	4	

Strength Training Program

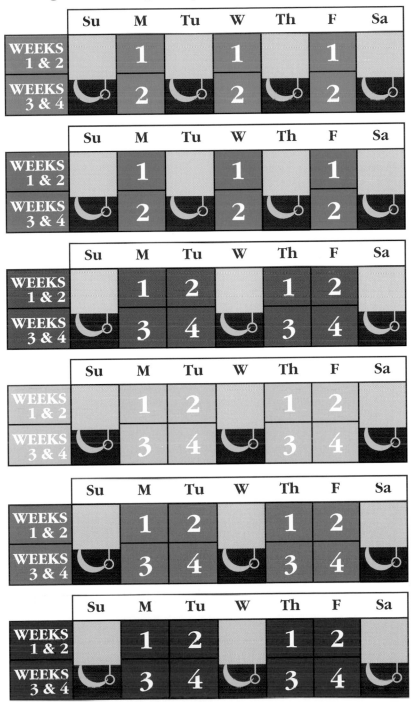

	Su	M	Tu	W	Th	F	Sa
WEEKS 1 & 2		1		1		1	
WEEKS 3 & 4		2		2		2	

	Su	M	Tu	W	Th	F	Sa
WEEKS 1 & 2		1		1		1	
WEEKS 3 & 4		2		2		2	

	Su	M	Tu	W	Th	F	Sa
WEEKS 1 & 2		1	2		1	2	
WEEKS 3 & 4		3	4		3	4	

	Su	M	Tu	W	Th	F	Sa
WEEKS 1 & 2		1	2		1	2	
WEEKS 3 & 4		3	4		3	4	

	Su	M	Tu	W	Th	F	Sa
WEEKS 1 & 2		1	2		1	2	
WEEKS 3 & 4		3	4		3	4	

	Su	M	Tu	W	Th	F	Sa
WEEKS 1 & 2		1	2		1	2	
WEEKS 3 & 4		3	4		3	4	

Cross-Training

After following your weight training program for several months, you may be getting bored with it. Rather than stopping your training, consider a cross-training program. Recall from chapter 1 that while weight training can improve the fitness components of muscular strength, endurance, body composition, and flexibility, its value in promoting cardiovascular fitness is minimal. By adding aerobic exercise to your weight workouts you can avoid boredom while improving your cardiovascular fitness level. The cross-training programs that follow will enable you to maintain the gains made from weight training while you improve your cardiovascular fitness levels and overall appearance.

Cross-Training for the Muscle Toning Program

To add cross-training workouts to your muscle toning program, include an aerobic exercise "interval" after every weight training set. The aerobic interval should consist of stair climbing, stationary cycling, jogging in place, jumping rope, or any other type of aerobic exercise that you can perform near the weight training exercise stations. The length of time in each aerobic exercise interval should be 30 seconds.

After the last repetition of each weight training set, begin immediately performing whatever aerobic exercise you have filled in on your workout chart. To maximize the benefits of a cross-training program, *do not delay the start of the aerobic interval.*

Cross-Training for the Body Shaping Program

To add cross-training to your body shaping program, add aerobic workouts on the nonweight training days; you will be exercising a total of 4 to 6 days per week. Although the body shaping workouts will develop your muscles and shape your body, adding aerobic exercise to your overall program will bring about a "sculpting" effect to your body much faster! Because aerobic exercise increases the number of calories being burned, adding aerobics to your overall program will reduce your body fat while the weight training builds up your muscles. The result of cross-training for you is a visually appealing physique. Many individuals choose to stair climb, stationary cycle, jog, run, walk, swim, or do aerobic dance two to three times per week on their days off from weight training. A sample cross-training program is provided on page 132. The number of aerobic exercise sessions you complete each week should be based on your weight training zone. If you are a beginner following the Green or Blue zone workouts, add 2 days of aerobic exercise per week. If you are an intermediate exerciser and use the Purple or Yellow body shaping workouts, you can do aerobic exercise 3 days per week. If you are more advanced and adhere to the Orange or Red zone workouts, you can also add three aerobic sessions per week. You will not need a special cross-training/weight training workout sheet; however, you may want to record the time, distance, type of exercise, and heart rate on a separate sheet to monitor your improvements.

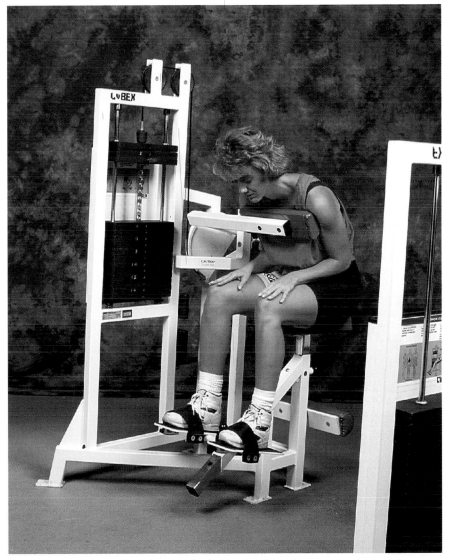

Aerobic exercise can complement the lighter loads and many repetitions of a muscle toning program.

Cross-Training for the Body Shaping Program

	Su	M	Tu	W	Th	F	Sa	Aerobic Interval
WEEKS 1 & 2		1	Run	1		1	Stair climb	Week 1: 15 min / Week 2: 17 min
WEEKS 3 & 4		2	Run	2		2	Stair climb	Week 3: 19 min / Week 4: 19 min

	Su	M	Tu	W	Th	F	Sa	Aerobic Interval
WEEKS 1 & 2		1	Aerobic dance	1		1	Cycle	Week 1: 21 min / Week 2: 23 min
WEEKS 3 & 4		2	Aerobic dance	2		2	Cycle	Week 3: 25 min / Week 4: 25 min

	Su	M	Tu	W	Th	F	Sa	Aerobic Interval
WEEKS 1 & 2		1	Run	1	Swim	1	Aerobic dance	Week 1: 25 min / Week 2: 27 min
WEEKS 3 & 4		2	Run	2	Swim	2	Aerobic dance	Week 3: 29 min / Week 4: 29 min

	Su	M	Tu	W	Th	F	Sa	Aerobic Interval
WEEKS 1 & 2	Stair climb	1	2	Run	1	2	Aerobic dance	Week 1: 31 min / Week 2: 33 min
WEEKS 3 & 4	Stair climb	3	4	Run	3	4	Aerobic dance	Week 3: 35 min / Week 4: 35 min

	Su	M	Tu	W	Th	F	Sa	Aerobic Interval
WEEKS 1 & 2	Run	1	2	Aerobic dance	1	2	Cycle	Week 1: 35 min / Week 2: 37 min
WEEKS 3 & 4	Run	3	4	Aerobic dance	3	4	Cycle	Week 3: 39 min / Week 4: 39 min

	Su	M	Tu	W	Th	F	Sa	Aerobic Interval
WEEKS 1 & 2	Swim	1	2	Stair climb	1	2	Run	Week 1: 41 min / Week 2: 43 min
WEEKS 3 & 4	Swim	3	4	Stair climb	3	4	Run	Week 3: 45 min / Week 4: 45 min

Cross-Training for the Strength Training Program

If you are serious about developing high levels of strength, you should not add aerobic exercise to a strength training program. Due to the heavier loads required to improve muscular strength, you need to rest properly; this not only applies to the period between sets and exercises but to the nonweight training days as well. If you attempt to incorporate aerobic exercise into a strength training program, you will find that you may not feel "recovered" or rested enough to complete the more intense weight training workouts; similarly, you may have to struggle through your aerobic workouts.

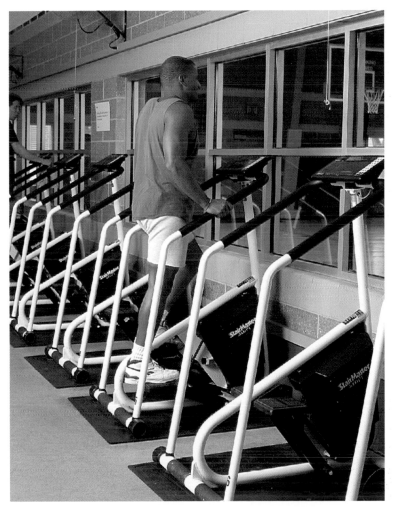

Increase the duration of your aerobic workouts gradually as you maintain or increase the intensity of your weight training workouts.

The Intensity of the Aerobic Component

To determine the intensity of an aerobic workout or interval, use your pulse or heart rate as a guide. The harder you exercise, the more your heart rate will increase. It is important to monitor your heart rate during aerobic exercise, because it helps you determine if you are exercising at a safe level yet hard enough to improve your cardiovascular fitness. Exercise can be dangerous if experienced at a level of intensity higher than what is recommended.

To determine your appropriate aerobic exercise intensity, follow these steps:

1. **Determine your *Maximum Heart Rate* (MHR).**
   Subtract your age from 220:

   $$220 - \text{your age} = \text{MHR (beats per minute)}$$

   220 – _____ (your age) = _____ your **MHR**

2. **Determine your *Target Heart Rate* (THR).**
   Your heart rate should fall within a range of 70% to 85% of your **MHR.** So, multiply your MHR by .70 and .85 to determine your **THR** range in beats per minute:

   MHR × .70 = **THR** (lowest value)

   _____ (your **MHR**) × .70 = _____ lowest **THR**

   MHR × .85 = **THR** (highest value)

   _____ (your **MHR**) × .85 = _____ highest **THR**

For example, if you're 30 years old, your MHR is 190 beats/minute:

$$220 - 30 = 190$$

And your target heart rate range is 133 to 161.5 beats/minute:

$$190 \times .70 = 133 \text{ (lower limit)}$$

$$190 \times .85 = 161.5 \text{ (upper limit)}$$

For a quick and accurate assessment of your heart rate during your aerobic workout or interval, take your heart rate within 10 seconds after exercising. Count your pulse for 10 seconds, then multiply by 6 or consult the following table.

Heart Rate Conversion Table	
Heart rate (per minute)	**Pulse rate** (10 seconds)
192	32
186	31
180	30
174	29
168	28
162	27
156	26
150	25
144	24
138	23
132	22
126	21
120	20
114	19
108	18
102	17
96	16
90	15

For example, if you felt 24 heartbeats in 10 seconds, your heart rate per minute would equal 144.

To take your heart rate during exercise, you can feel or "palpate" your pulse on several places on your body. The most effective locations are at the radial artery on the thumb side of your wrist and at the carotid artery just below your jaw on the neck.

At the end of each aerobic interval or during your aerobic workout, simply look at your wristwatch or wall clock, place your fingers at either pulse rate location, and count your heart rate for 10 seconds. Your goal is to reach but not to exceed your 10-second THR range. If your pulse rate is too high, then step, pedal, jog, or jump rope more slowly. If your pulse is too low, then increase your intensity.

The Duration of the Aerobic Component

For the muscle toning program, the duration of your aerobic portion is the rest period between your weight training sets (30 seconds). When following a body shaping cross-training program, the duration is longer. Beginners can perform 15 to 25 minutes of aerobic exercise per session.

Intermediates can aerobically exercise 25 to 35 minutes, and advanced persons can complete 35 to 45 minutes of aerobic exercise per session. Be aware that these are only guidelines; for example, even if you are in the Purple zone, it does not mean that you have to run for 30 minutes each workout, even though you may have never run that far before. If you feel that the aerobic workouts are too difficult, move back to a lower level and increase your duration gradually.

14

Charting Your Progress

Earlier in this book you were asked to think generally about your goals to help you decide between muscle toning, body shaping, or strength training programs. Here, we'll challenge you to consider goals that are more specific. In the last section of this chapter we provide some "keys" to successful training that will make your training safer and more effective.

Determining What You Really Want Out of Training

If you haven't yet given serious consideration to what you want specifically from your training, you will find the following series of questions helpful in developing short-term and long-term goals and in finding ways to chart your progress toward them.

Consider which of the following goals you would like to attain:

- **Fitness goals**
  Do you want to increase your muscle endurance? Increase your strength? Recover from workouts faster? Improve your cardiovascular endurance?

- **Personal appearance goals**
  Do you want to tone your muscles? Fit into your clothes better? Gain muscle and lose fat?
- **Personal goals**
  Do you want to improve your energy level? Improve how you see yourself?
- **Activity goals**
  Do you want to improve performance in a specific sport? Improve your abilities in recreational activities?

After considering these long-term goals, establish some weight training goals that can be either short (3 months) or long (1 or more years) term. Consider the following ideas when formulating your training goals, and establish time lines for each.

- **Workout goals**
  Do you want to increase loads? Increase sets? In which exercises?
- **Cardiovascular goals** (for programs including aerobic exercise)
  Do you want a lower heart rate at rest? The ability to recover more quickly from a workout? The ability to complete greater distances or to assume a greater workload (bicycle, rowing machines) during workouts of the same length?

These goals, combined with the information written in the workout chart, will help you assess your progress as you weight train. Use this list to start thinking about your personal goals for weight training. You may not seek improvements in all the areas listed above; you may want to work toward goals that are even more specific. If you follow the weight training programs outlined in this book, you should easily advance toward any goals you may have.

Keys to Successful Training

As you weight train, remember to keep these keys in mind.

Train on a Regular Basis

You are virtually guaranteed success if you follow the workouts presented in chapters 6 through 11—which means you will be training on a regular basis. *Sporadic training does not produce results!*

Gradually Increase Workout Intensity

Gradually increasing the intensity of training allows your muscles to adjust to strenuous workouts and then to improve their tone, endurance, size, and strength. The workouts included in this book are developed with this principle in mind.

Don't Underestimate the Importance of Nutrition and Rest

Remember the training equation:

$$\frac{\text{Regular}}{\text{training}} + \frac{\text{Balanced}}{\text{meals}} + \frac{\text{Adequate}}{\text{rest}} = \frac{\text{Dramatic}}{\text{improvements}}$$

If one of the three factors is absent, your outcomes will be less than optimal. While much has been written on the value of nutritional supplements—especially those high in protein—respected nutritionists continue to stress that balanced meals (12% protein, 58% carbohydrates and 30% fat) provide our nutritional needs, including protein. A good source of nutritional information can be found in *Nancy Clark's Sports Nutrition Guidebook*.

In addition to nutrition, your body needs rest to rebuild muscles after training as much as it needs training to stimulate muscle growth. Initially, you need to train two or three times a week. More is not always better,

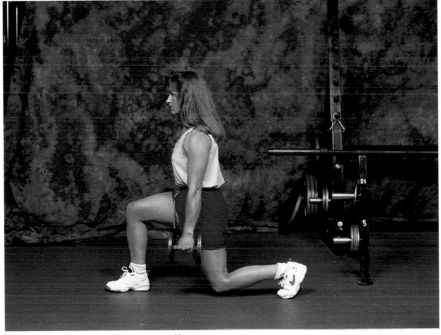

Remember, preseverence pays off.

because training too often doesn't allow enough time for your muscles to receive nutrition and to rebuild, and it may actually result in a *loss* of muscle tissue. Training smart means you train on a regular basis, eat balanced meals, and get enough rest. This fact cannot be overemphasized.

Develop and Maintain a Positive Attitude

Nothing worthwhile comes easily. You have to believe that weight training can produce dramatic improvements in your appearance, fitness status, and physical performance—and it does! Get psyched, because you're in for a treat! Every minute, every day makes a difference! Admittedly, training is uncomfortable at times, but perseverance pays off. The "burn" hurts, but that burn is what molds your body, helps reduce body fat, and accentuates muscle tone. Do not miss one training session; one leads to two, two to three, and then what you could have achieved will not happen. Develop the attitude that the hour you put aside for training is the time you are doing something for yourself. It's *your* time, so be selfish with it. In the end you'll feel better about yourself; you'll be more productive in your life, and you'll be healthier. It's the one thing you can do in an hour that will positively impact your appearance, fitness status, health, and physical performance. Your investment in training time will be richly rewarded!

Appendix A

Exercises Illustrated

The following pages illustrate correct movement technique for the exercises contained in the workouts in Part II. The exercises are arranged according to the muscle group they work and the type of exercise they are [free weight (FW), pivot machine (PM), and cam machine (CM) exercises]. The first figure is the initial or start position and the second figure shows the action by way of movement arrows. Closed arrowheads indicate the movement direction, open arrowheads indicate the direction of the return movement. In exercises for which a spotter is recommended, the spotter's role in the action is illustrated.

Abdomen

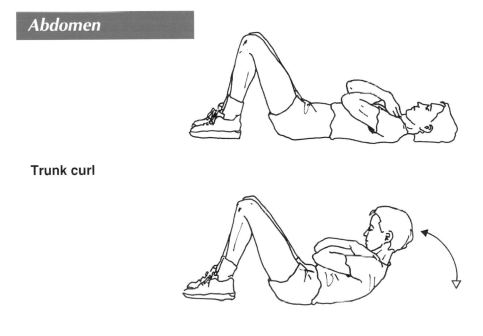

Trunk curl

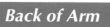

CM
Trunk curl

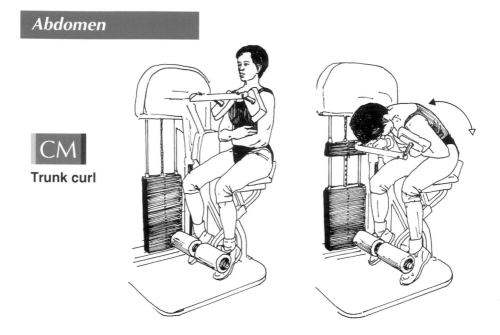

Back of Arm

FW
Triceps extension

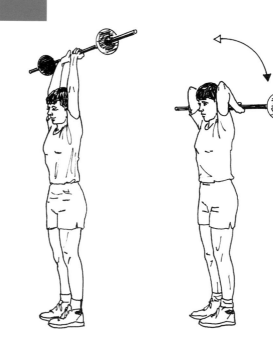

Back of Arm

**Triceps
push-down**

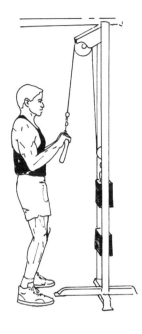

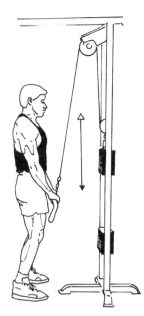

**Triceps
extension**

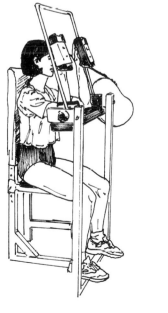

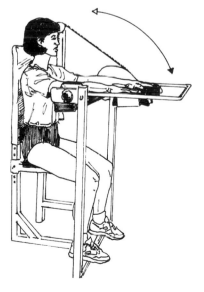

Front of Arm

FW

Biceps curl

PM

Low pulley curl

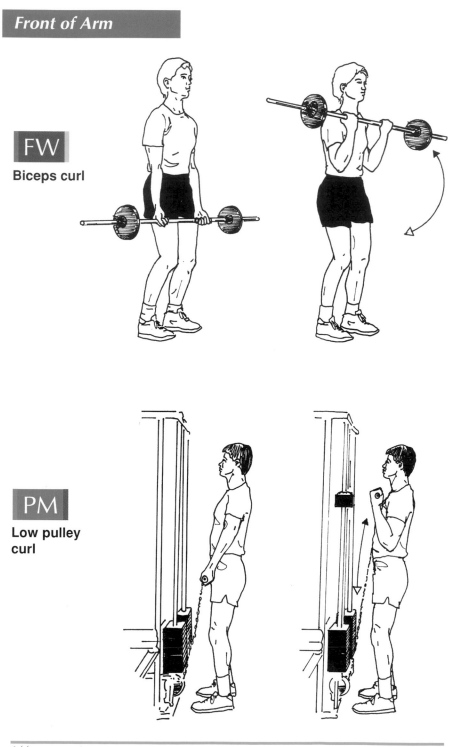

144

Front of Arm

Preacher curl

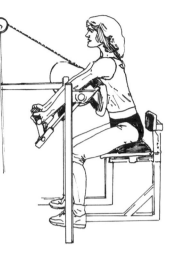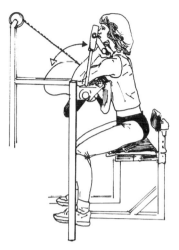

Back

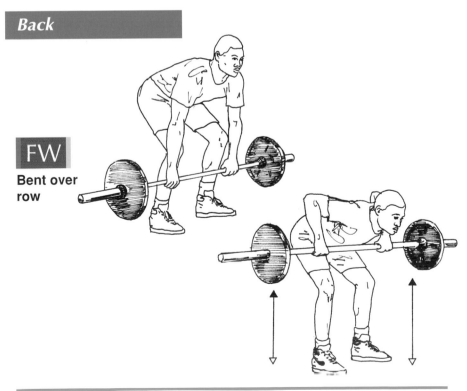

FW
Bent over row

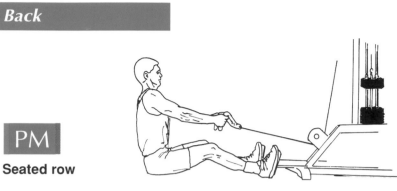

Seated row

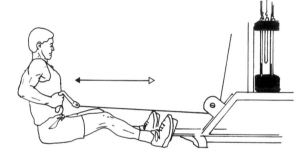

**Rowing
exercise**

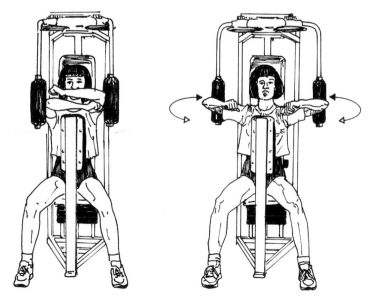

Back

Dumbbell Row

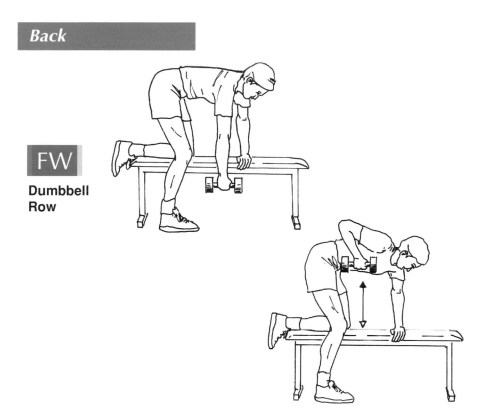

Lat pull-down

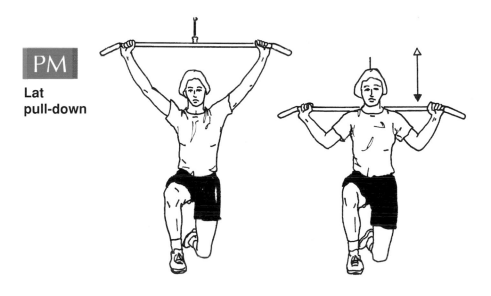

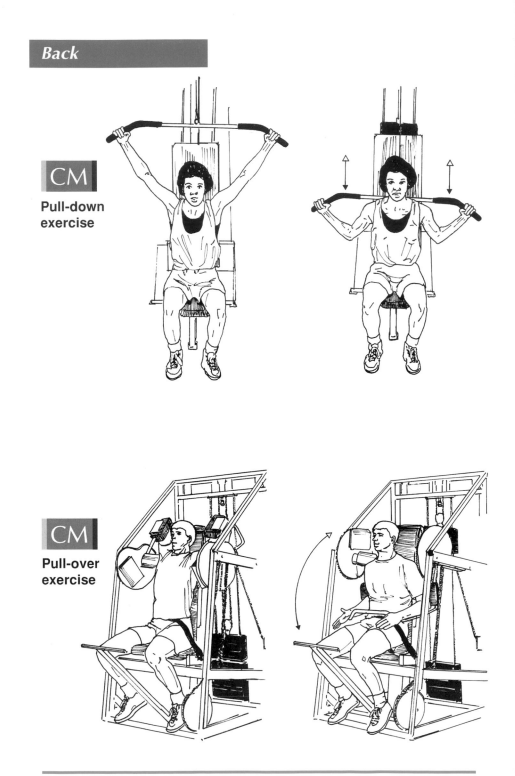

CM

Pull-down exercise

CM

Pull-over exercise

Calf

FW

Standing calf raise

PM

Heel raise

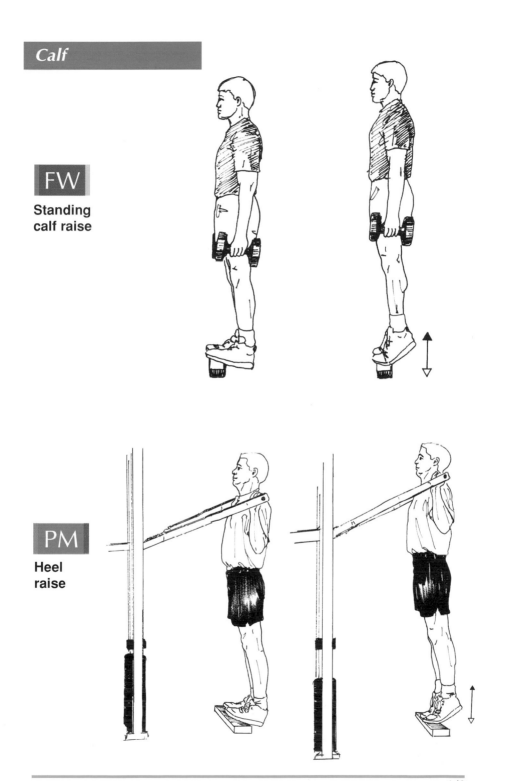

Calf

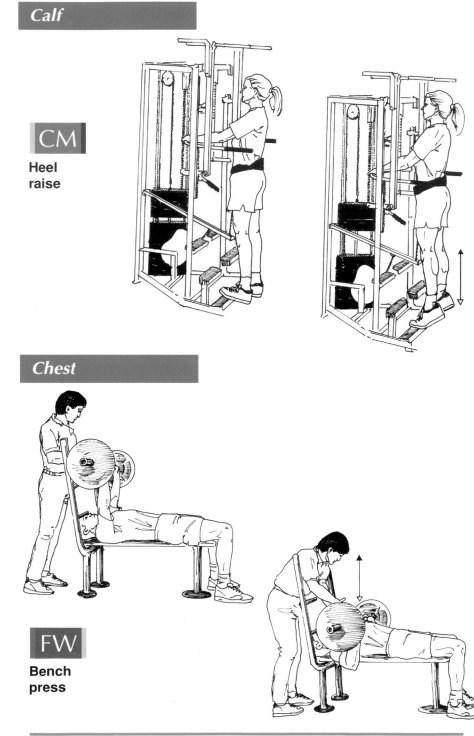

CM

Heel raise

Chest

FW

Bench press

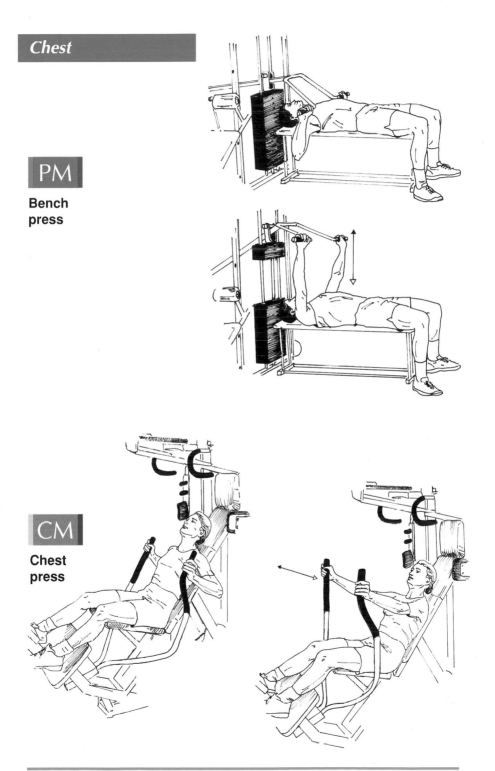

Chest

PM

Bench press

CM

Chest press

Chest

**Dumbbell
fly**

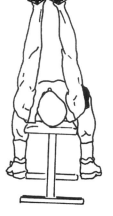

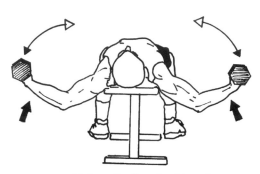

Note: *Spotter should spot wrists at points indicated by thick arrows.*

**Pec deck
(butterfly)**

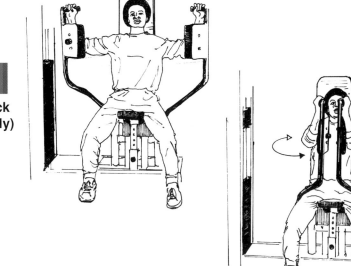

Chest

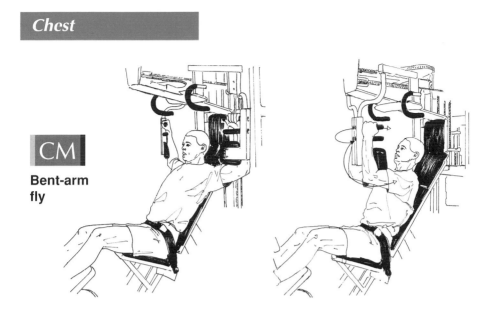

CM

Bent-arm fly

Shoulder

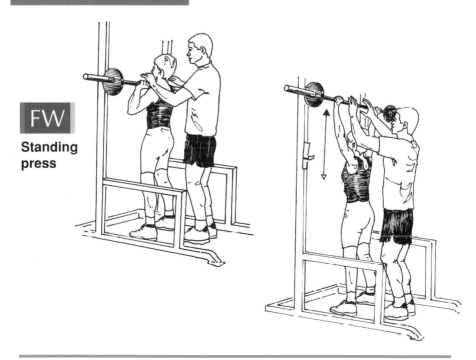

FW

Standing press

Shoulder

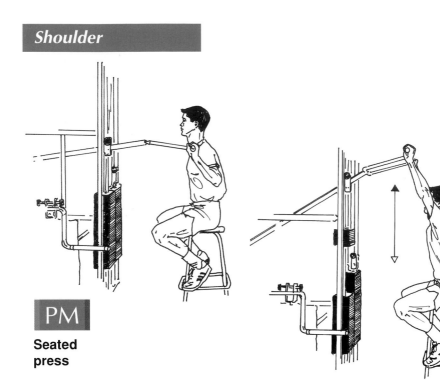

PM

**Seated
press**

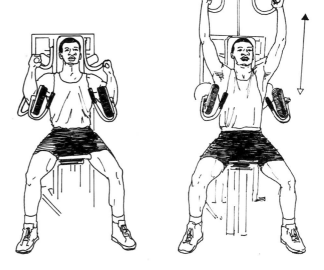

CM

**Shoulder
press**

Back of Thigh

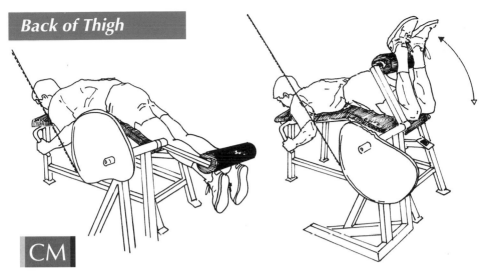

CM

Leg curl

Note: *Movement patterns for this exercise are identical on a pivot machine.*

Front of Thigh

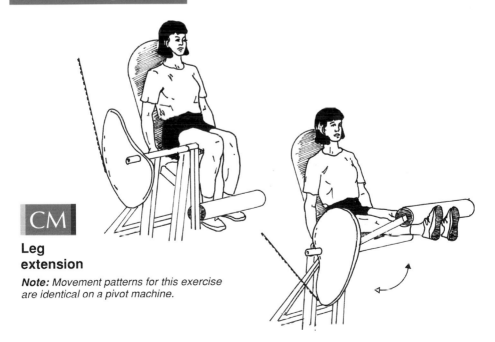

CM

Leg extension

Note: *Movement patterns for this exercise are identical on a pivot machine.*

Thigh

FW

Lunge

FW

Squats

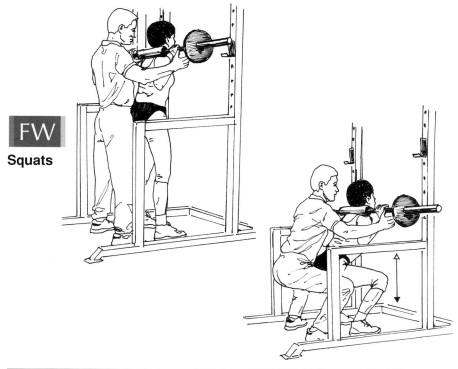

Thigh

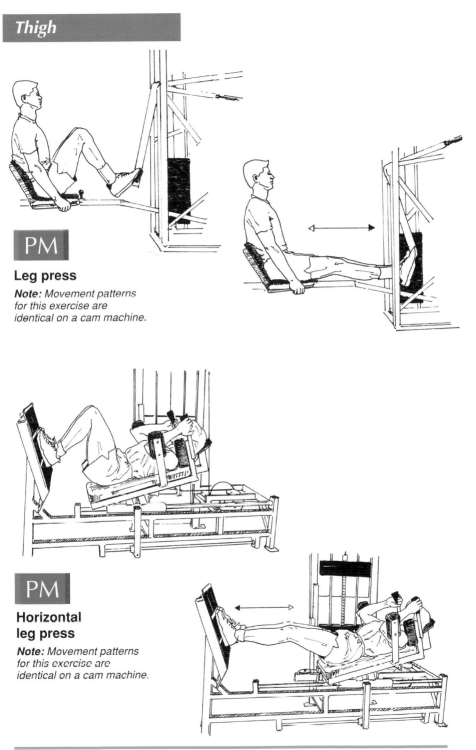

PM

Leg press

Note: Movement patterns for this exercise are identical on a cam machine.

PM

Horizontal leg press

Note: Movement patterns for this exercise are identical on a cam machine.

Thigh

CM

Dual leg press

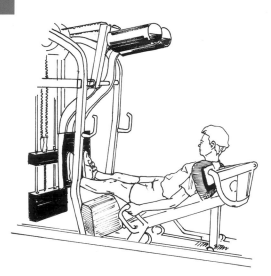

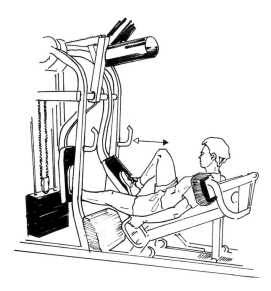

Workout Charts

Weight Training 2 Days/Week

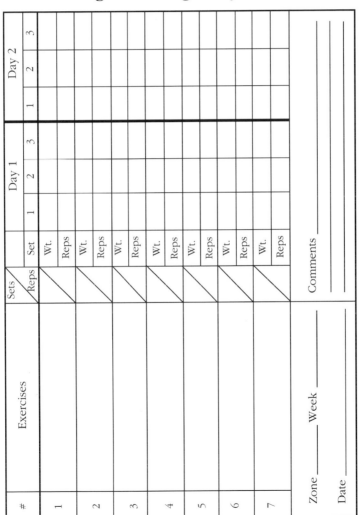

#	Exercises	Sets		Set	Day 1			Day 2		
		Reps			1	2	3	1	2	3
1				Wt.						
				Reps						
2				Wt.						
				Reps						
3				Wt.						
				Reps						
4				Wt.						
				Reps						
5				Wt.						
				Reps						
6				Wt.						
				Reps						
7				Wt.						
				Reps						

Zone _____ Week _____

Date _____

Comments _____

Weight Training 3 Days/Week

#	Exercises	Sets Reps	Set	Day 1 1	2	3	4	Day 2 1	2	3	4	Day 3 1	2	3	4
1			Wt.												
			Reps												
2			Wt.												
			Reps												
3			Wt.												
			Reps												
4			Wt.												
			Reps												
5			Wt.												
			Reps												
6			Wt.												
			Reps												
7			Wt.												
			Reps												
8			Wt.												
			Reps												
9			Wt.												
			Reps												
10			Wt.												
			Reps												

Comments

Zone _____ Week _____

Date _____

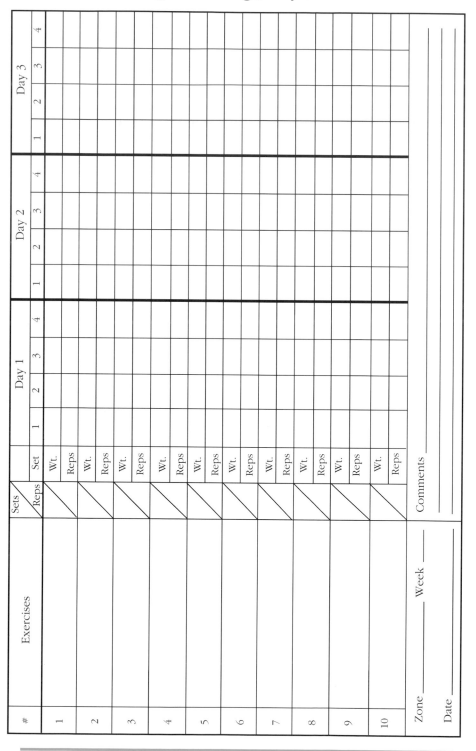

Weight Training 4 Days/Week

#	Upper body exercises	Sets/Reps	Set	Day 1				Day 3			
				1	2	3	4	1	2	3	4
1			Wt.								
			Reps								
2			Wt.								
			Reps								
3			Wt.								
			Reps								
4			Wt.								
			Reps								
5			Wt.								
			Reps								
6			Wt.								
			Reps								
7			Wt.								
			Reps								

#	Lower body exercises	Sets/Reps	Set	Day 2				Day 4			
				1	2	3	4	1	2	3	4
1			Wt.								
			Reps								
2			Wt.								
			Reps								
3			Wt.								
			Reps								
4			Wt.								
			Reps								
5			Wt.								
			Reps								
6			Wt.								
			Reps								

Zone _____ Week _____

Date _____

Comments _____
_____
_____

Cross-Training 3 Days/Week

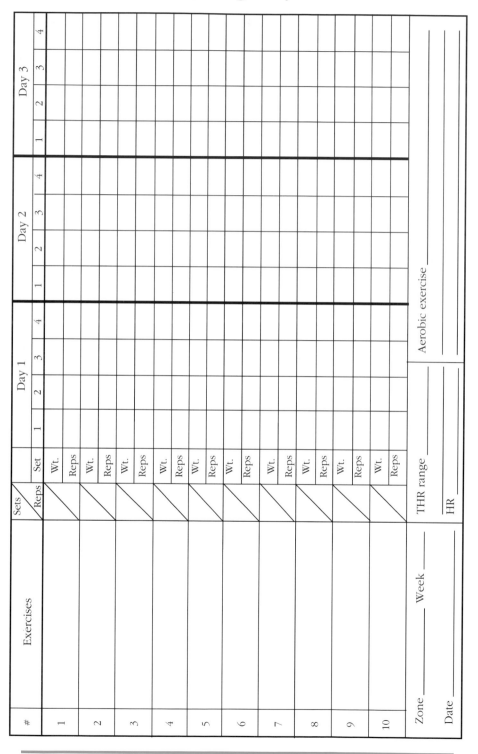

#	Exercises	Sets		Set	Day 1				Day 2				Day 3			
			Reps		1	2	3	4	1	2	3	4	1	2	3	4
1				Wt.												
				Reps												
2				Wt.												
				Reps												
3				Wt.												
				Reps												
4				Wt.												
				Reps												
5				Wt.												
				Reps												
6				Wt.												
				Reps												
7				Wt.												
				Reps												
8				Wt.												
				Reps												
9				Wt.												
				Reps												
10				Wt.												
				Reps												

Zone _____ Week _____

Date _____

THR range _____

HR _____

Aerobic exercise _____

Cross-Training 4 Days/Week

#	Upper body exercises	Sets / Reps	Set	Day 1				Day 3			
				1	2	3	4	1	2	3	4
1			Wt.								
			Reps								
2			Wt.								
			Reps								
3			Wt.								
			Reps								
4			Wt.								
			Reps								
5			Wt.								
			Reps								
6			Wt.								
			Reps								
7			Wt.								
			Reps								

#	Lower body exercises	Sets / Reps	Set	Day 2				Day 4			
				1	2	3	4	1	2	3	4
1			Wt.								
			Reps								
2			Wt.								
			Reps								
3			Wt.								
			Reps								
4			Wt.								
			Reps								
5			Wt.								
			Reps								
6			Wt.								
			Reps								

Zone_____ Week_____

Date_____

THR range_____

HR _____

Aerobic exercise _____

_____

_____

References

Baechle, T.R. (Ed.) (1994). *Essentials of Strength Training and Conditioning*. National Strength and Conditioning Association. Champaign, IL: Human Kinetics.

Baechle, T.R., & Earle, R. (1989). *Weight training: A text for the college student*. Omaha: Creighton University.

Baechle, T.R., & Groves, B.R. (1992). *Weight training: Steps to success*. Champaign, IL: Human Kinetics.

Baechle, T.R., & Groves, B.R. (1993). *Weight training video* [videotape]. Champaign, IL: Human Kinetics.

Baechle, T.R., & Groves, B.R. (1994). *Weight training instruction*. Champaign, IL: Human Kinetics.

Clark, N. (1990). *Nancy Clark's sports nutrition guidebook*. Champaign, IL: Human Kinetics.

Fleck, S., & Kraemer, W. (1987). *Designing resistance training programs*. Champaign, IL: Human Kinetics.

Garhammer, J. (1986). *Sports Illustrated strength training*. New York: Harper & Row.

Getchell, B. (1983). *Physical fitness: A way of life* (3rd ed.). New York: Wiley.

Hoeger, W.K. (1989). *Lifetime fitness, physical fitness and wellness* (2nd ed.). Englewood, CO: Morton.

Holloway, J., & Baechle, T.R. (1990). Strength training for female athletes. *Sports Medicine*, **9** (4), 216-228.

Kraemer, W., & Baechle, T.R. (1989). Development of a strength training program. In J. Ryan & F.L. Allman, Jr. (Eds.), *Sports medicine* (2nd ed.) (pp. 113-127). San Diego, CA: Academic Press.

Lombardi, V.P. (1989). *Beginning weight training: The safe and effective way*. Dubuque, IA: W.C. Brown.

O'Shea, J.P. (1976). *Scientific principles and methods of strength fitness*. Menlo Park, CA: Addison-Wesley.

Stone, M., & O'Bryant, H. (1987). *Weight training: A scientific approach*. Minneapolis: Burgess.

Index

Sets
    determining number of, 122, 124
    recording of, 110
Shoes, 15
Shoulder press, 154
Shoulders
    stretching exercises for, 36, 37
    weight training exercises for, 153-154
Squats, 156
Standing calf raise, 149
Standing press, 153
Storage of equipment, 33
Strength training
    blue zone workouts for, 54, 59-60
    cross-training with, 133
    definition of, 5
    green zone workouts for, 45, 51-52
    orange zone workouts for, 84, 91-94
    purple zone workouts for, 62, 67-70
    red zone workouts for, 96, 103-106
    training schedule for, 129
    yellow zone workouts for, 72, 79-82
Stretching exercises, 36-39
    for arms, 37
    for back, 37, 38, 39
    basic guidelines, 36
    for calves, 39
    for chest, 36
    for hamstrings, 39
    for hips, 38
    for quadriceps, 38
    for shoulders, 36, 37
    for triceps, 37
Success, keys to, 138-140
Supportive equipment, 16-17, 31

T
Thighs, strength training exercises for
    for back of thigh, 155
    for front of thigh, 155
    leg curl, 155
    leg extension, 155
    leg presses, 157-158
    lunge, 156
    squats, 156
Trainers, personal, 20
Training goals, 41-42, 120, 137-138
Training heart rate (THR), 134
Training load. See Load, determination of
Training logs (workout charts), 109-111, 138, 159-163
Training program design. See Program design

Training schedules
    basic guidelines, 126, 138
    for blue zone workouts, 54
    for body shaping program, 128
    for green zone workouts, 46
    for muscle toning program, 127
    for orange zone workouts, 84
    for purple zone workouts, 62
    for red zone workouts, 96
    for strength training program, 129
    for yellow zone workouts, 72
Training success, keys to, 138-140
Triceps
    stretching exercises for, 37
    weight training exercises for, 142, 143
Trunk curl, 141-142
2-for-2 rule, 120

W
Warming up
    basic guidelines, 35
    stretching exercises for, 36-39
Weight belts, 16, 31
Workout charts (logs), 109-111, 138, 159-163
Workout goals, 138. See also Goal setting
Workout zones
    basic explanation of, 41, 43
    blue zone, 53-60
    color-coding of, 41
    green zone, 45-52
    how to choose, 42
    orange zone, 83-94
    purple zone, 61-70
    red zone, 95-106
    yellow zone, 71-82
Wraps, 17
Wrist wraps, 17

Y
Yellow zone workouts, 71-82
    basic guidelines, 71-72
    for body shaping, 71-72, 75-78
    load determination for, 115-120, 121
    for muscle toning, 71, 73-74
    for strength training, 72, 79-82
    training schedule for, 72

About
the Authors

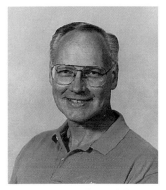
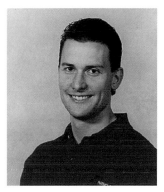

Thomas Baechle   **Roger Earle**

Thomas R. Baechle, EdD, CSCS, is the executive director of the Certified Strength and Conditioning Specialists Agency, the certifying body for the National Strength and Conditioning Association (NSCA). He is co-founder and past president of NSCA, former Director of Education, and in 1985 was named their Strength and Conditioning Professional of the Year. Dr. Baechle is also the chair of the Department of Exercise Sciences and the exercise leader of the Phase III Cardiac Rehabilitation Program at Creighton University in Omaha, where he has received several honors, including an Excellence in Teaching Award.

Dr. Baechle holds certifications as a Level I weightlifting coach from the United States Weightlifting Federation, a Strength and Conditioning Specialist and Personal Trainer from NSCA, and an Exercise Test Technologist and Exercise Specialist from the American College of Sports Medicine (ACSM). He has authored several texts, including *Weight Training: Steps to Success*, and has published more than 30 articles on the topic of weight and strength training.

Roger W. Earle, MA, CSCS, earned his master's degree in exercise science from the University of Nebraska at Omaha. He is the head strength and conditioning coach and is on the faculty of the Department of Exercise Science at Creighton University. In addition, he has served as a personal fitness trainer for individuals at all age and fitness levels for nearly 10 years. Earle serves as the Nebraska State Director of NSCA. He is certified as a Strength and Conditioning Specialist and Personal Trainer by NSCA and as a Health and Fitness Instructor by ACSM.

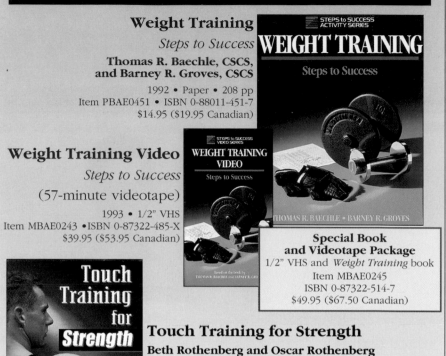